PRACTICAL ECHOCARDIOGRAPHY IN THE ADULT
with Doppler and color-Doppler flow imaging

Developments in Cardiovascular Medicine

VOLUME 109

PRACTICAL ECHOCARDIOGRAPHY IN THE ADULT

with Doppler and color-Doppler flow imaging

by

J.P.M. HAMER

Thoraxcentre, Department of Cardiology,
University Hospital Groningen,
Groningen,
The Netherlands

KLUWER ACADEMIC PUBLISHERS

DORDRECHT / BOSTON / LONDON

Library of Congress Cataloging-in-Publication Data

Hamer, J. P. M.
    Practical echocardiography in the adult : with Doppler and color
Doppler flow imaging / by J.P.M. Hamer.
        p.   cm. -- (Developments in cardiovascular medicine ; v. 109)
    ISBN-13:978-94-010-6734-8   e-ISBN-13:978-94-009-0549-8
    DOI: 10.1007/978-94-009-0549-8

    1. Doppler echocardiography.   2. Transesophageal echocardiography.
3. Heart--Diseases--Diagnosis.   I. Title.   II. Series.
    [DNLM: 1. Echocardiography, Doppler--in adulthood.   2. Heart
Diseases--diagnosis.   3. Heart Diseases--in adulthood.   W1 DE997VME
v. 109 / WG 141.5.E2 H214P]
    RC683.5.U5H35   1990
    616.1'207543--dc20
    DNLM/DLC
    for Library of Congress   90-4146
ISBN-13:978-94-010-6734-8

Published by Kluwer Academic Publishers,
P.O. Box 17, 3300 AA Dordrecht, The Netherlands

Kluwer Academic Publishers incorporates
the publishing programmes of
D. Reidel, Martinus Nijhoff, Dr W. Junk and MTP Press.

Sold and distributed in the U.S.A. and Canada
by Kluwer Academic Publishers,
101 Philip Drive, Norwell, MA 02061, U.S.A.

In all other countries, sold and distributed
by Kluwer Academic Publishers Group,
P.O. Box 322, 3300 AH dordrecht, The Netherlands

printed on acid free paper

Contents

Foreword

Since the introduction of ultrasound in cardiology in the mid fifties, echocardiography has continued to grow and has finally become, in particular after the introduction of Doppler modalities, the working horse of the cardiologist.

Although many books have been written on this subject Dr. Hamer's book is a very valuable contribution, as it provides, in particular information for practicing clinicians and technicians. Clearly written and nicely illustrated, this book is a must for those interested in this field.

C.A. Visser
Professor of Echocardiology

Preface

Trans-thoracic echocardiography is a patient friendly technique without pain or discomfort. It is harmless and the patient can relax during the examination. With these advantages in mind there is hardly any technique in cardiology that can provide so much valuable information about the function of the heart.

If Doppler and color Doppler, also painless techniques, are added to echocardiography additional information about blood flow velocities, insufficiency and stenosis of valves, detection of shunts etc. is obtainable.

Less patient friendly but – if selectively used – very informative, is trans-esophageal (color Doppler) echocardiography.

Echocardiography is a sophisticated technique giving the investigator a great responsibility. If used properly, the result of the investigation nearly always has clinical implications. Therefore the role of the technician in the treatment of the patient may also be important. The aim of the technique is not only to obtain measurements from some standard positions since conclusions often have to be drawn without the support of measurements. The observed motion patterns of the heart and valves can sometimes be more important for the evaluation of the severity of an abnormality than a certain number of millimeters. It is the investigators responsibility to make correct measurements and to express the visual impressions in order to make an accurate report which adequately describes the severity of the disorder.

The aim of this book is to explain echocardiography and Doppler, and to answer questions concerning their use. This has been achieved by supplementing the text with drawings, photographs and Doppler illustrations.

The principles of echocardiography, Doppler, color Doppler and trans-esophageal echocardiography are discussed with standard transducer positions and the technically optimal methods for making recordings. Special attention has been paid to anticipating and answering the most common questions. In addition, phonocardiography and pulse recording are discussed briefly.

For specific abnormalities, obligatory investigations with echocardiography, Doppler and/or pulse recordings can be found in the sections entitled 'to be investigated in . . .'. When necessary, a brief differential diagnosis is given in the sections entitled 'to be excluded'.

A diagnosis can be made from two points of view: from specific recordings, or from the point of view of a specific heart disease. This book handles the problems from both perspectives. The anatomy, nomenclature and function of the normal heart are described separately as background information for the technician. Also, the echo- and Doppler findings in specific heart diseases are preceded by a short description of the disease.

Several books could be filled with all the possible measurements from the echo- and phonocardiogram. For practical reasons, only those measurements which are practically and clinically useful and which are used by the majority of institutions, are presented here.

It may be that all the techniques (echo, echo-Doppler and color Doppler, trans-esophageal echocardiography, phonocardiography and pulse recording) are useful in the diagnosis and estimation of the severity of cardiac disorders. The clinical applications of each modality are mentioned for various cardiac disorders with the most important transducer positions. The most important rules are mentioned, as are the exceptions and the pitfalls.

It is not possible in a book of this format to cover all the details of cardiac disease. Very rare cardiac or extracardiac disorders are not discussed: for this, several excellent works are available. The short and deliberately practical approach which is presented here, should cover most situations and any limitations are due to the selection that had to be made.

Acknowledgements

I would like to acknowledge Boehringer Ingelheim Alkmaar for their permission to reproduce Figures 2-3 to 2-5, 2-7, 2-9, 2-11, 2-15, 2-17 and 6-11 and Toshiba Medical Systems Europe for their permission to reproduce Figures 3-3 to 3-11 and 6-10.

Also, I would like to thank Toshiba Medical Systems Europe for their kind cooperation and for their excellent equipment which made it possible to obtain almost all the recordings for this book.

Especially, I thank Mrs Biddy Schilizzi for correcting the text.

Chapter 1. Principles of ultrasound

Introduction

The use of ultrasound for the detection of structures, their motion patterns and their distances from the observer is not only related to echography; it is older than mankind and well known from the world of animals. The dolphin and the bat, for example, use it for exploring their environment and finding directions.

The same principle is used in geography for calculating the depth of the sea and the layers in the earth's crust.

For medical purposes ultrasound was used, a long time ago, to localize the mid-brain. In the early fifties the mitral valve was visualized for the first time with ultrasound, but it took many years before the technique was clinically available.

Ultrasound is – by definition – inaudible with a frequency of more than 20.000 Hz. For echocardiography much higher frequencies are used, from 1 to 11 MegaHerz that is 1 11 million Herz. For trans thoracic echocardiographic examinations frequencies from 2-5 MHz are normally used, depending on the situation.

The basic unit of ultrasound is a piezo-electrical crystal. It has the property of producing soundwaves if activated by an electrical impulse. Conversely, if such a crystal is hit by proper sound waves, it produces an electrical current.

For ultrasound examinations, one or a series of piezo electric crystals are used. When activated electrically they function as a transmitter (producer of ultrasound), when activated by reflected ultrasound they produce an electrical current and function as a receiver. As both functions are alternately used in the same crystal, the unit is called a transducer.

If a transducer is electrically activated for a short period it causes an ultrasound impulse of short duration. This impulse needs a certain time to reach a certain depth; the same time is needed for the reflected ultrasound to return to the transducer. The sum of these times is converted by the machine into a certain distance on a monitor. Accordingly, a distance can be measured only when a pulsed system is used. The measurement is only correct if the machine is calibrated for the velocity of ultrasound in the medium through which the ultrasound passes, which is 1,540 m/sec for blood and about the same for soft tissues. A machine that is calibrated for this velocity will calculate a distance incorrectly if the medium is bone or air: the velocity through air is much lower and through bone much higher than through blood and soft tissues.

Terminology

An echo can be projected on a monitor as a vertical deflection from a baseline. The more powerful the echo is, the larger is the amplitude of the deflection. This is called the Amplitude-mode or A-mode (Fig. 1-1).

Instead of a large amplitude, a powerful echo can also be represented by a bright dot, and a weak echo by a less bright dot: this is called the Brightness mode or B-mode. When a strip of light-sensitive paper is drawn over the dots of a B-mode image, the motion of a dot will be recorded as a motion on the paper. This is called the Motion-mode or M-mode (Fig. 1-1).

When structures with different acoustical impedances (different interfaces) are situated behind each other, the line that represents the ultrasound beam from one crystal shows a series of B-mode dots behind each other.

When more crystals are used in one transducer, each crystal can be represented by one line. Since these lines are arranged divergently in one plane, a sector is visible on the screen, which is a B-mode image. This two-dimensional (2D) image shows the anatomy and events of the heart in one specific plane.

One specific line can be chosen from the sector image to obtain an M-mode recording. This line is called the M-line (Fig. 1-2).

If two M-mode recordings are made simultaneously with help of two M-lines, the recording is called a dual M-mode recording. An M-mode sweep or M-mode scan is obtained if the M-line is moved through the sector image during M-mode recording. M-mode recordings are usually made at a speed of 50 mm/sec, M-mode sweeps at 25 mm/sec. If time-calculations have to be made, a paper speed of 100 mm/sec is advisable.

Types of systems

A sector image can be produced mechanically or electronically. There are advantages and disadvantages with both systems with respect to each other. The mechanical systems consist of a number of rotating crystals. The electron-

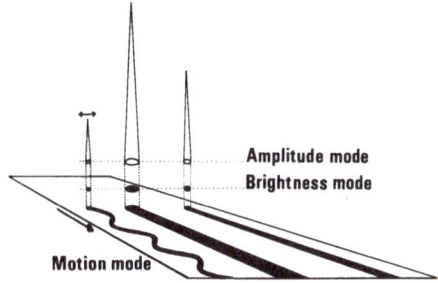

Fig. 1-1. Schematic representation of the possibilities of recording echoes. A powerful echo (such as the middle one) can be represented by a large vertical deflection, i.e. a large amplitude (Amplitude mode). A less powerful echo is represented by a deflection of smaller amplitude (right). These amplitudes can be converted into respectively a bright and a less bright dot (Brightness mode). An M-mode recording is obtained by projecting the motion of the B-mode dots on moving light-sensitive paper (Motion mode).

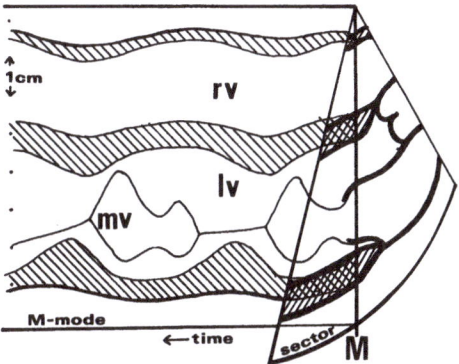

Fig. 1-2. Schematic representation of a sector image with an M-line (M) from which the M-mode recording is obtained. mv = mitral valve.

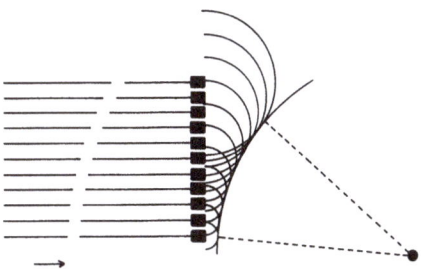

Fig. 1-3. A simplified representation of the method used to obtain a specific focus in a phased array system. Each interruption in the horizontal lines represents the moment of activation of the crystals. If the sequential pulsing is made as shown, a certain focus of the transducer is obtained. The focus can be changed easily by modification to the pulsing sequence.

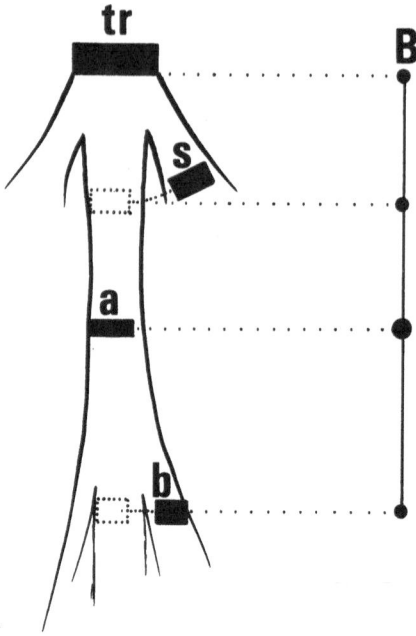

Fig. 1-4. Diagram illustrating the problem of lateral resolution. The ultrasound beam from the transducer (tr) hits structure 'a' which is found in the midline of the ultrasound beam. Consequently, the echo from 'a' will be projected correctly on the B-line that represents the middle of the ultrasound beam. The divergent properties of the ultrasound beam, mean that structure 'b' also reflects the ultrasound. This echo is 'seen' by the transducer as originating from the midline and will be falsely projected on the B-line. The same is possible for structures in side lobes ('s').

ically or phased array systems have a number of small crystals, from which the timing of activation is steered electronically

Image quality

The ultrasound beam

Frequency of the transducer. One of the factors that influence the quality of the echo-image is the transducer frequency. A low frequency has a good penetration in depth as only a few interfaces will reflect the ultrasound and much ultrasound remains available for further penetration; the resolution (the ability to distinguish objects that are close together) however, is worse. On the other hand, a high frequency transducer has a poor penetration in depth but a better resolution. So, the frequency of the transducer to be selected, depends on the requirements. For imaging the first few centimeters, higher frequencies

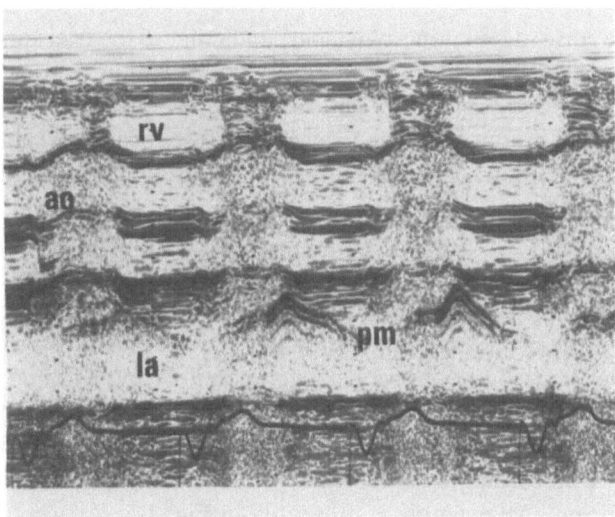

Fig. 1-5. Left parasternal M-mode recording. In the left atrium (la) behind the aorta (ao), echoes from a pacemaker wire, present in the right atrium, are falsely projected in the posterior aortic wall and in the left atrium. This is caused by the divergent character of the ultrasound beam. The machine recognizes these echoes as coming from the midline of the ultrasound beam.

are required: for pediatric echocardiography and for trans-esophageal echocardiography 5-7 MHz is often advisable. For trans-thoracic adult echocardiography lower frequencies from 2-4 MHz have to be used.

Focus. An ultrasound beam is divergent. The distance from the transducer at which the divergency starts depends on the size of the transducer and its frequency. The more divergency, the worse the echo-picture will be. There are various methods for focussing transducers at different depths to obtain a focal zone for that area in which the investigator is specifically interested.

Electronic focussing in a phased array system is schematically shown in Fig. 1-3.

Axial resolution. Axial resolution expresses the ability to distinguish objects that are close together and arranged along the axis of the transducer. Axial resolution is strongly related to the transducer frequency. Two or more objects that are present in one wavelength are identified as only one object. To distinguish such objects, a short wavelength is needed. For example, with a 3.75 MHz transducer, objects closer than 0.4 mm to each other can not be distinguished.

Lateral resolution. Lateral resolution expresses the ability to distinguish objects that are close together in a plane perpendicular to the transducer. Lateral resolution is equal to the beam diameter. Objects within the beam diameter will not be identified separately, but recognized as one object in which case lateral resolution is poor. Further away (behind the focal zone) lateral resolution worsens as the ultrasound beam diverges (Fig. 1-4). Part of this problem can be solved by focussing the ultrasound beam at a deeper level.

Side lobes. One of the problems of the ultrasound beam is the presence of side lobes. Side lobes strike objects that are positioned near to and lateral from the transducer. If the ultrasound is reflected from such objects towards the transducer, the echoes will not be recognized as coming from a lateral area. They are 'projected' on a line through the middle of the ultrasound beam (Fig.1-4).

Consequently, structures behind or in front of the plane of section can be seen on the echocardiogram, due to side lobes and the divergency of the ultrasound beam. An example is presented in Fig. 1-5: a pacemaker wire is located in the right atrium.

However, in this long axis view the echoes from the pacemaker wire are projected in the left atrium and the posterior aortic wall. This is caused by the strongly reflecting wire, so that even the weak echoes from the divergent part of the ultrasound beam are reflected. These echoes are not recognized by the machine as coming from outside the midline of the ultrasound beam.

This specific example will not raise problems in the interpretation of the echocardiogram. However, other poorly recognizable structures may be confusing.

Reverberations. When an ultrasound beam strikes an object, it is reflected towards the transducer. However, the transducer can function as a reflecting object for those echoes, especially if the echoes are powerful (Fig. 1-6).

The transducer reflects the echoes, and the ultrasound hits the object a second time. The object again reflects the ultrasound towards the transducer. These transmissions take twice the normal time. From the first echoes, the echo-system locates the object at a correct distance. However, the second echoes (reverberations) are projected at twice the distance from the transducer.

The transducer is not the only reflecting structure to produce reverberations. Every intracardiac structure can cause this phenomenon, such as the mitral leaflets (Fig. 1-7).

The usually strong echoes returning from the pericardium reach the transducer and the distance from the transducer is identified. Part of the ultrasound however, is reflected by the atrial surface of the anterior mitral leaflet and returns towards the pericardium; the echoes are reflected again towards the transducer. They reach the transducer a short time later. As time is distance,

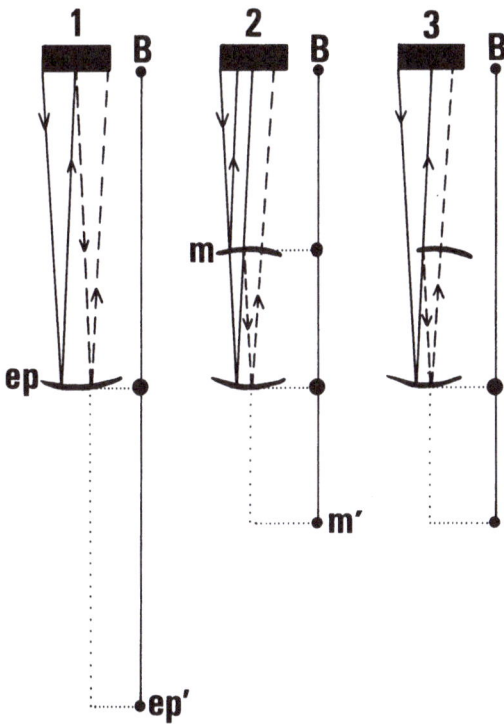

Fig. 1-6. Schematic representation of causes of reverberations. At 1 the ultrasound is reflected by the epicardium and projects it correctly on the B-line. However, the transducer itself functions as a reflecting structure, causing a false echo from the epicardium at a double distance from the transducer (ep').

At 2 the echoes from the epicardium that cross the mitral valve (m) are partly reflected by the valve, then by the epicardium and then return to the transducer; this causes a second projection (mirror image) m' of the mitral valve behind the heart (Fig. 1-7).

At 3 the mitral valve is hit only by the echoes that return from the epicardium; they reflect against the valve and than return to the transducer. This explains why a mirror image projection of the mitral valve can be found behind the heart without projection of the mitral valve in the LV (Fig. 1-7).

the echo-system projects these echoes at a greater distance from the transducer. Consequently, a mirror-image of the anterior mitral leaflet is projected behind the pericardium. Reverberations are also illustrated in Fig. 1-8; it shows that the direction of the reflected ultrasound is not necessarily in line with the transducer: the mitral valve is not visible in the correctly projected echocardiogram, but only as a reverberation behind the heart.

These examples of reverberation do not lead to misinterpretation of the echocardiogram. However, other structures may cause confusing reverberations in the heart itself.

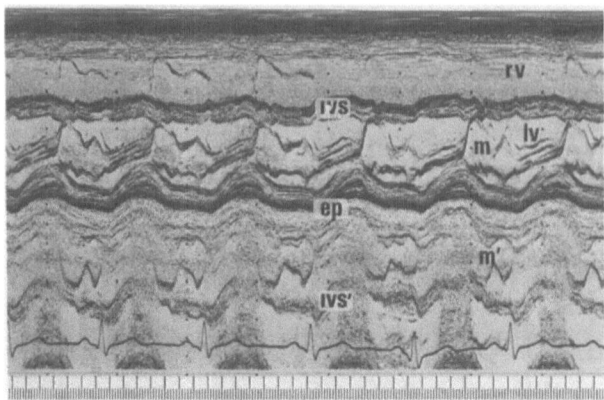

Fig. 1-7. Left parasternal M-mode recording with reverberations caused by the strongly reflecting epicardium. Mirror images of the mitral valve (m') and of the IVS (ivs') are projected behind the heart (see also Fig. 1-6).

Strong reverberations are also caused by prosthetic valves (Fig. 1-9) by the disc and by surrounding structures. These are very disturbing as they 'shield' echoes from structures behind the prosthetic valves.

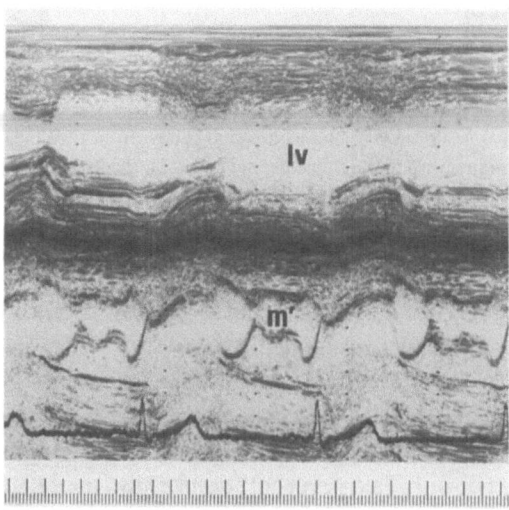

Fig. 1-8. Projection of the echoes of mitral leaflets (m') behind the heart without visible mitral leaflets in the lv. See Fig. 1-6 for explanation.

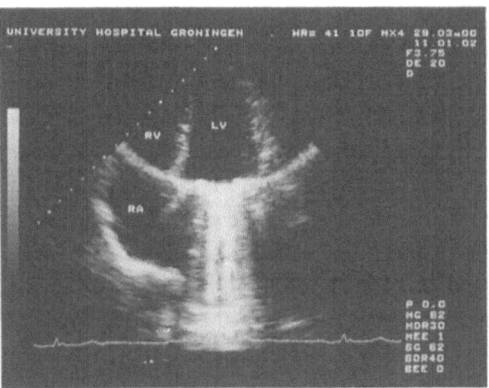

Fig. 1-9. Apical view of a mechanical mitral valve prosthesis. The prosthesis causes strong reverberations, shielding the left atrium.

The medium

Ultrasound travels through a medium and reflects from each layer with a different 'acoustical impedance'. The greater the difference in acoustical impedance, the more ultrasound will be reflected. In case of very great acoustical impedances, hardly any or no ultrasound passes the interface. This is well known from echocardiograms from prosthetic valves. The valve itself may cause strong reverberations and structures behind it cannot be visualized (Fig. 1-9).

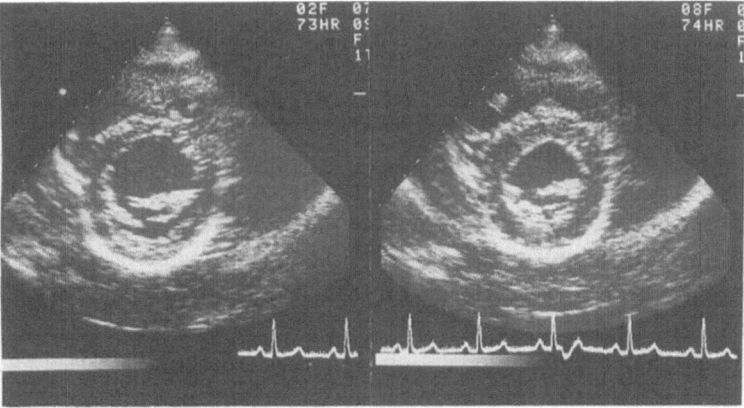

Fig. 1-10. Short axis view of the left ventricle during diastole (left) and systole. Particularly in the diastolic frame, 'defects' can be seen in the myocardium. This is partly caused by the angle between the ultrasound beams and the surface of the septal and lateral parts of the LV. Echoes are much better from structures that are (almost) perpendicular to the transducer.

Ultrasound looses its power with increasing distance from the transducer. This loss of power not only depends on the differences in acoustical impedances but also on the properties of the medium. The power will be maintained for a long time in pure water, but is rapidly diminished in blood and still more in muscle. Air nearly totally absorbs ultrasound which explains the impossibilty of obtaining echocardiograms if there is air-containing lung tissue between transducer and heart. Consequently, a good echocardiogram can rarely be obtained from an obese patient with emphysema.

The power of an echo also depends on the angle between the surface of the object and the ultrasound beam. This is illustrated in Fig. 1-10: a good image in this short axis view of the LV is obtained from the anterior and posterior part; the weakest echoes are from the septum and the lateral wall.

Ultrasound is reflected by the septum and the lateral wall, not only because the inner surface of the LV is not totally smooth, but also because of scattering of ultrasound: very small irregularities of a surface reflect ultrasound in all directions (angle independent!) and some of these echoes will be directed towards the transducer.

Manipulation of echoes

Gain control. The power of echoes depends on many factors and differs between individuals. It is necessary to have a means of varying the overall intensity of echoes. This is accomplished with the overall gain control. Also, as ultrasound has much power in the near field and will loose its power when it travels through a medium, the capability to suppress echoes from the near field and enhance echoes from the far field is needed. This can be done with every echo-machine with the segmental gain control for various levels from the transducer. For each investigation new gain settings are necessary. It is advisable to start an examination with a high gain setting in order to detect small, weak echoes (Fig. 1-11). Echo-empty areas, like blood containing compartments, should show some 'snow'.

Reject control. The valuable information that can be obtained from echoes is usually mixed with information that disturbs the image and/or interpretation. Small, irrelevant echoes are always present and have to be rejected as much as possible. For this, the reject control is used. The more rejection, the higher the level below which the echoes disappear. Large echoes however, remain as large as they are. This differs from the gain control: a lower gain setting reduces all echoes.

Gray scale. A gray scale is good when bright weak echoes are visible in varying shades of gray. Without a gray scale the picture is only black and white. The

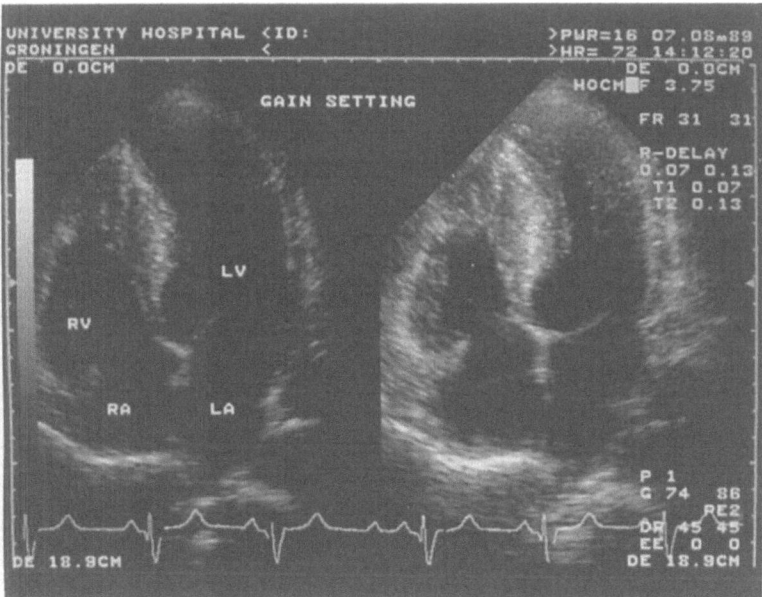

Fig. 1-11. Apical view of HCM, illustrating the importance of correct gain setting. With a low gain setting (left) many structures are identified, but with a higher gain setting the unexpected position of the ventricular endocardium can be identified.

better the gray scale, the wider the dynamic range. The dynamic range -expressed in decibels- is the ability of the system to record available signals: the range of valuable echoes. The more decibels in the dynamic range, the better the gray scale. This control is not important when recording normal valves, but is extremely valuable for the quality of recordings of other structures e.g. myocardium, valve vegetations, intracavitary echo-masses etc.

References

Edler I: Ultrasound cardiogram in mitral valve disease. Acta Chir Scand 111:230, 1956.

Wells PNT: Physics: An introduction to echocardiography. Edited by G.Leech and G.Sutton. London, Medi-Cine Ltd., 1978.

Eggleton RC: Interim AIUM Standard Nomenclature. Reflections 4:275, 1978.

Yeh E: Reverberations in echocardiograms. J Clin Ultrasound 5:84, 1977.

Feigenbaum H: Safety of diagnostic ultrasound. Ind State Med J 76:472, 1983.

Edler I, Gustafson A, Karlefors T, Christensson B: Ultrasound cardiography. Acta Med Scand (Suppl) 370:68, 1961.

Henry WL *et al.*: Report of the American Society of Echocardiography Committee on Nomenclature and Standards in Two-Dimensional Echocardiography. Circulation 62:212, 1980.

Chapter 2. Trans-thoracic echocardiographic examination

Position of the patient, examiner and equipment

Air-containing lung tissue prevents ultrasound penetration. Thus, it can be very difficult or impossible to obtain recordings from patients with emphysema. The area on the chest without lung tissue between the transducer and the heart is rather small. Usually this 'acoustic window' is only found from the lower left parasternal region to the apex. An abdominal acoustic window for examination of the heart and also for the IVC is the subcostal position. For examination of the thoracic aorta the suprasternal transducer position is useful.

With the patient lying at 90° on the left side, a rather large acoustic window is obtained. To make the acoustic window as large as possible, the patients left upper arm should be under the level of the left shoulder and the right lower arm leans on the patients lower trunk; head and spine should be bent forward a little. This is the best position to start the examination.

With the patient in this position it is almost always possible to obtain an image from the left parasternal region. For the apical transducer position the patient can, if necessary, be rotated a little to the right. The patient is supine for subcostal and suprasternal examinations.

In most institutions, both equipment and examiner are located on the right side of the patient. Echocardiographs have control panels that can be manipulated from both sides, but it is often more covenient with the left hand.

Echocardiographic examinations are sometimes very time-consuming and demand a lot of patience from the doctor as well as from the patient. With this in mind, the examiner should take a comfortable position. In this respect, the examiners chair and the height of the table are important. The table should be low, lower than most tables that are commercially available. The examiner should have an easy chair without armrests and adjustable in height; generally a high position is best. Also, most echocardiographs have the control panel at a

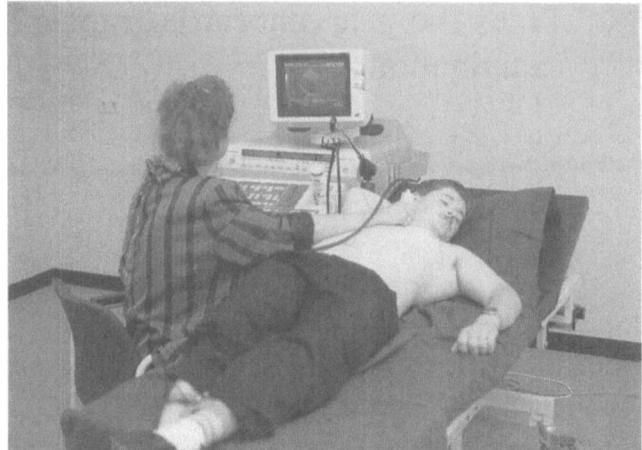

Fig. 2-1. The wrong position for echocardiographic examination: the chair has no wheels and is too low. The table is too high. The patient is not lying far enough on his left side and has his left upper arm above the shoulders.

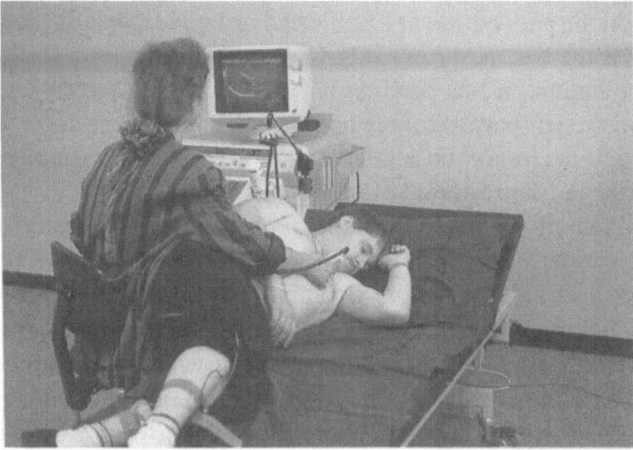

Fig. 2-2. Correct position for echocardiographic examination: a chair on wheels, the examiner at a higher position, the table lower, the patient lying more on his left side with the upper arms below the level of the shoulders.

rather high level and a high chair position makes using of the control panel easier. With the examiner and the table in these positions, the examiner can keep the right arm with the transducer at a low position and can often support the lower arm on the patients abdomen. This is less tiring for the examiner's shoulder. With the transducer held like a pencil, the right hand can lean on the patients chest (Fig. 2-1, 2-2).

Standard transducer positions

To obtain as much information as possible from the heart and its function, different transducer positions have to be used. The standard positions will be discussed but variations of these are also possible. For every examination it is advisable to make echocardiograms from at least all the standard positions.

The long axis view. To obtain the long axis view, the transducer is placed in the third or fourth intercostal space on the left side of the sternum. The sector plane is directed from the apex of the heart to the right shoulder (Fig. 2-3, 2-5, 2-6). A standard long axis view is obtained if the following structures are visible in one plane: part of the right ventricle, the aortic valve, the mitral valve, the LA and the greatest length and width of the LV; the IVS is hit perpendicularly by the ultrasound. Rather often a moderator band can be found in the RV.

This position is suitable for the evaluation of the LV, the IVS, the LVPW, the left atrium, the mitral valve, the aortic valve and the aortic root.

The short axis view of the ventricles. With the transducer in the same position as in the long axis view, but turned clockwise 90°, the short axis view of the ventricles is obtained (Fig. 2-4, 2-7, 2-8). The normal LV is recorded then as a circular structure, the RV hanging partly around it. Transverse sections can be made through the LV at the level of the mitral valve, the chordae tendineae and the papillary muscles.

This position is especially suitable for the evaluation of the motion pattern of the left ventricular wall.

The short axis view of the aorta. Often the transducer can be kept in the same place as in the short axis view of the ventricles to obtain the short axis view of the aorta (Fig. 2-4, 2-9, 2-10). The transducer is angled a little into the direction of the right shoulder. The sector plane then passes the outflow tract of the LV transversely and ends in the circular shaped aortic valve ring with the closure lines of the cusps. The closure line between right and non coronary cusp is the clearest one, as the ultrasound hits only this line perpendicularly. The pulmon-

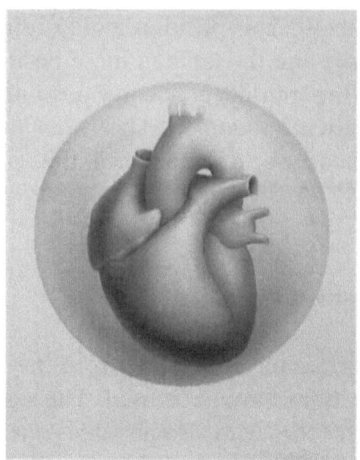

Fig. 2-3. Schematic representation of the heart as used to illustrate the cross sections for the long axis view (Fig. 2-5 and 2-6), the apical view (Fig. 2-11 and 2-12A, 2-12B), the subcostal view (Fig. 2-13 and 2-14) and the suprasternal view (Fig. 2-17 and 2-18).

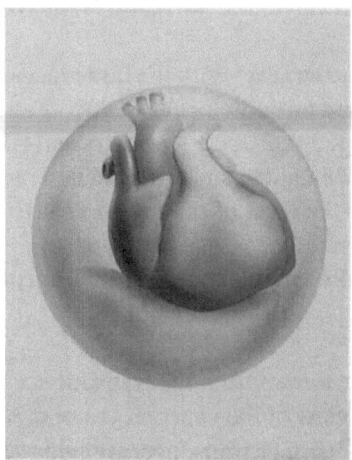

Fig. 2-4. Schematic representation of the heart as used to illustrate the cross sections for the short axis view of the ventricles (Fig. 2-7 and 2-8), the short axis view of the aorta (Fig. 2-9 and 2-10) and the IVC view (Fig. 2-15 and 2-16).

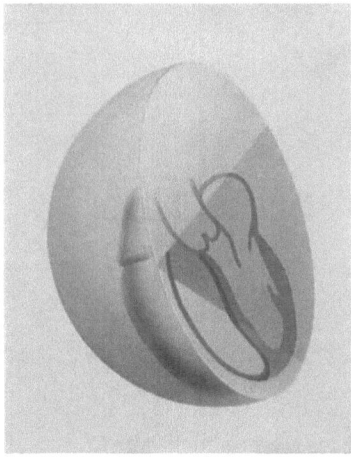

Fig. 2-5. Schematic representation of the long axis view as derived from Fig. 2-3.

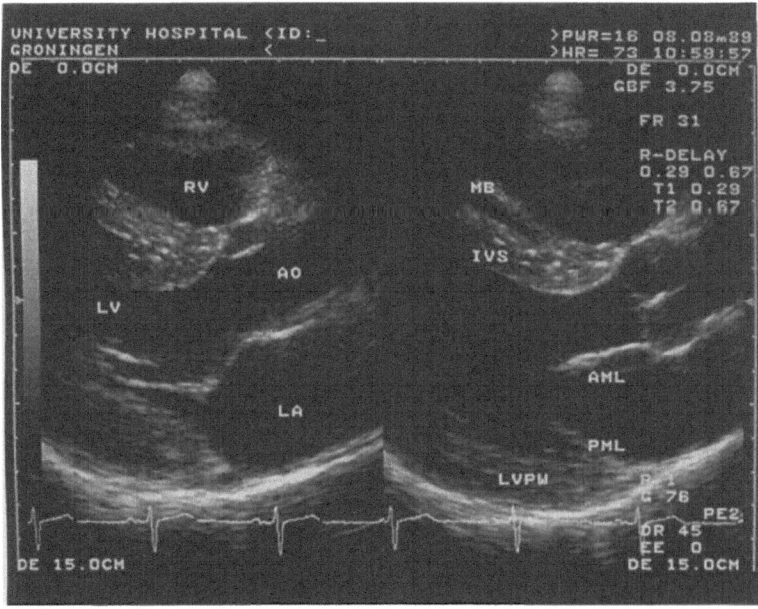

Fig. 2-6. A normal long axis view during diastole and systole. AO = aorta, MB = moderator band.

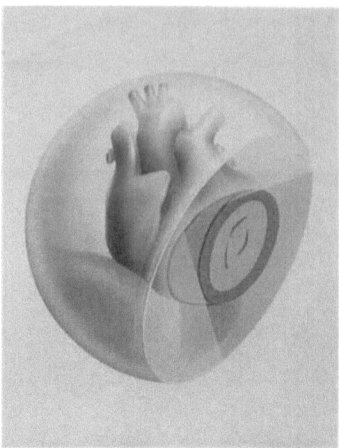

Fig. 2-7. Schematic representation of the short axis view of the ventricles as derived from Fig. 2-4.

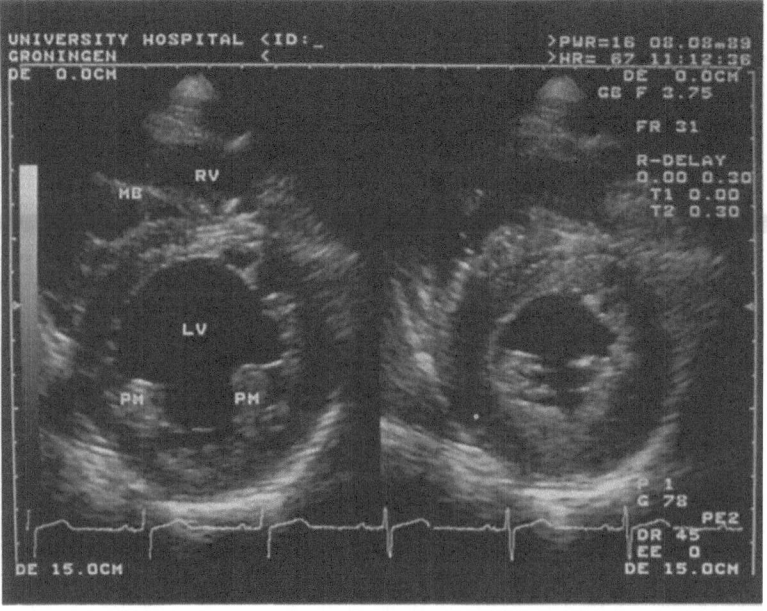

Fig. 2-8. A normal short axis view of the ventricles during diastole and systole. MB = moderator band, PM = papillary muscles.

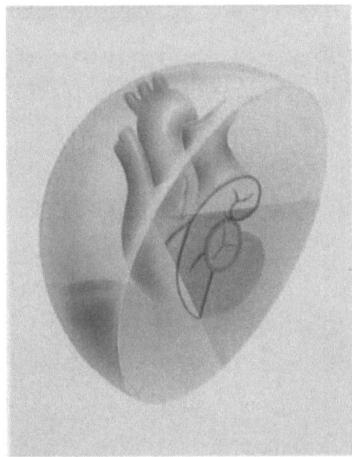

Fig. 2-9. Schematic representation of the short axis view of the aorta as derived from Fig. 2-4.

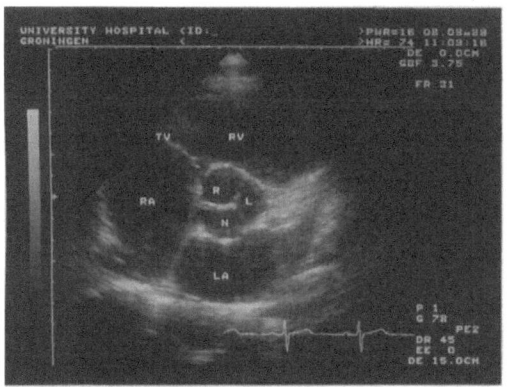

Fig. 2-10. A normal short axis view of the aorta. R = right coronary cusp, N = non coronary cusp, L = left coronary cusp, TV = tricuspid valve.

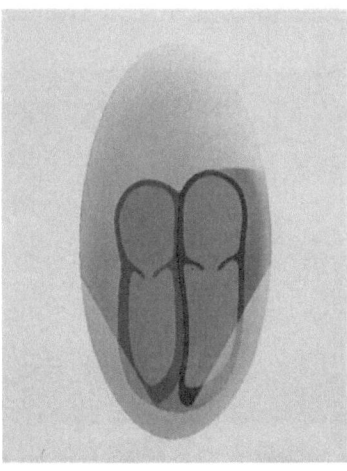

Fig. 2-11. Schematic representation of the apical (4 chamber) view as derived from Fig. 2-3.

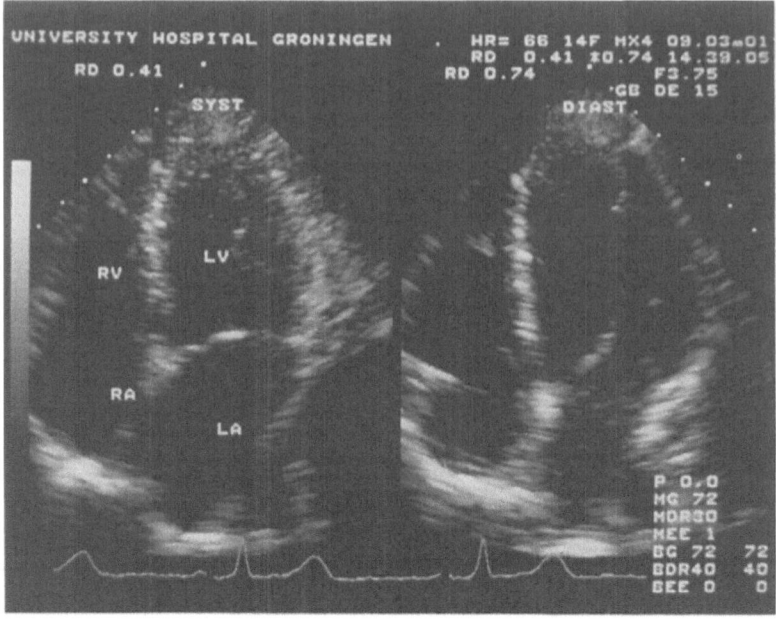

Fig. 2-12A. A normal 4 chamber apical view during systole and diastole.

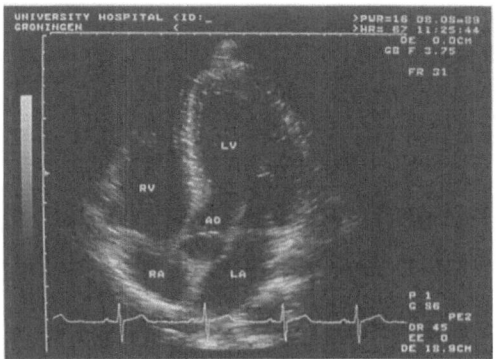

Fig. 2-12B. A normal 5 chamber apical view. AO = aorta.

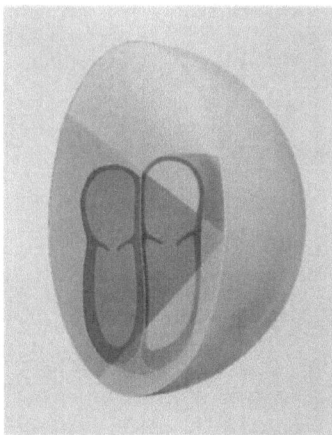

Fig. 2-13. Schematic representation of the subcostal view as derived from Fig. 2-3.

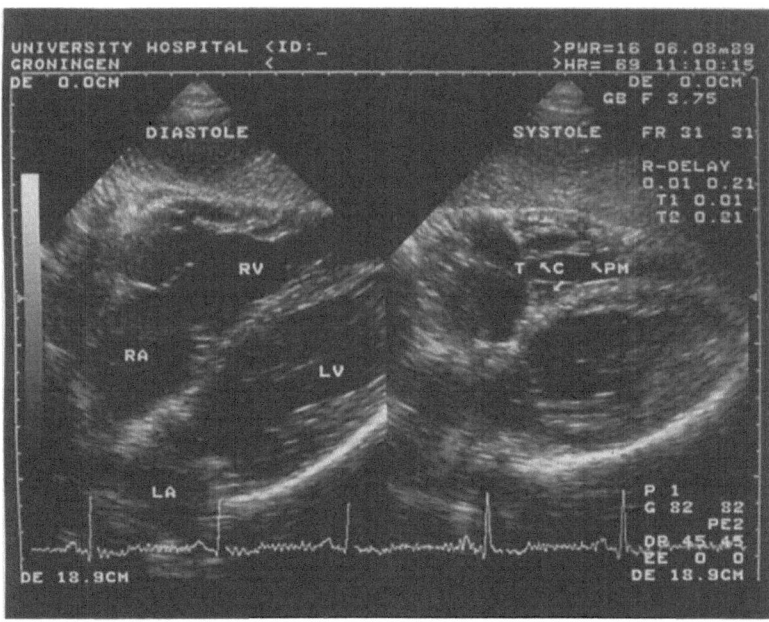

Fig. 2-14. A normal subcostal view during systole and diastole. T = tricuspid valve, PM = papillary muscle of tricuspid valve, C = chordae of tricuspid valve.

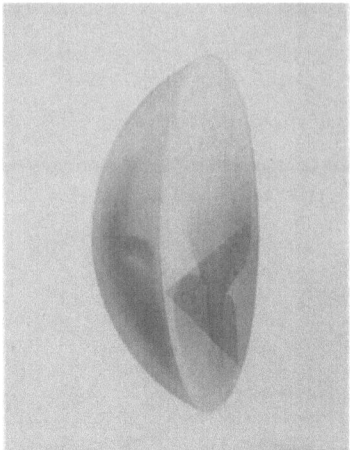

Fig. 2-15. Schematic representation of the IVC view as derived from Fig. 2-4.

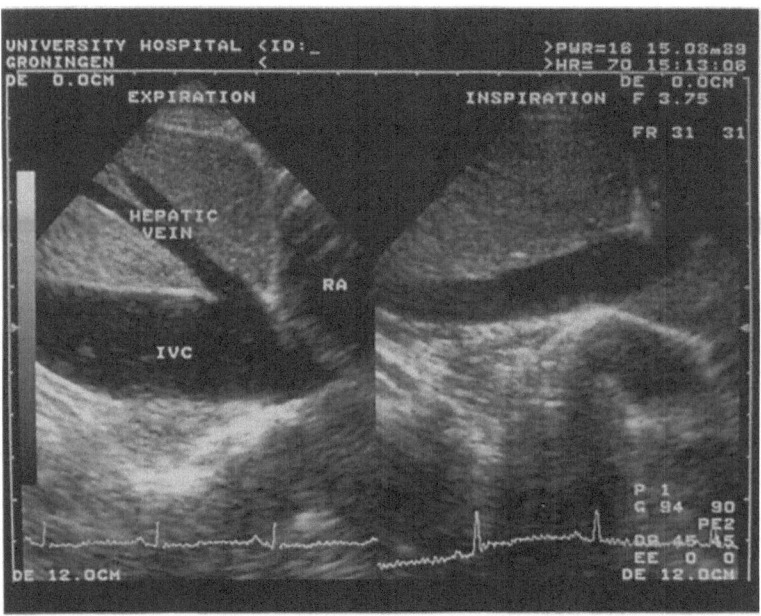

Fig. 2-16. A normal IVC view during respiration. The IVC collapses during inspiration, indicating a normal RA pressure.

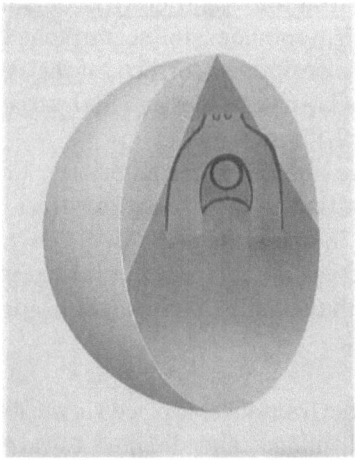

Fig. 2-17. Schematic representation of the suprasternal view as derived from Fig. 2-3.

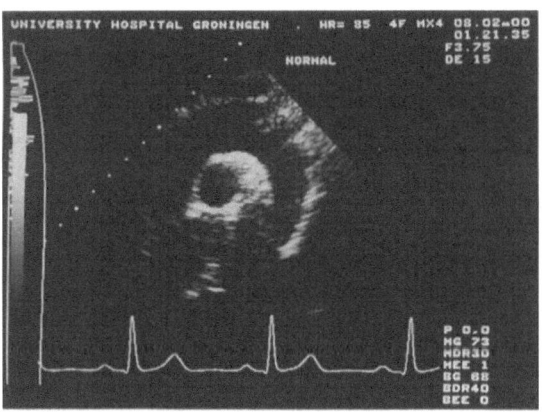

Fig. 2-18. A normal suprasternal view. The ascending aorta is on the left, the descending aorta on the right. The circular structure in the middle is a transverse section through the right pulmonary artery, below which the LA is recorded.

ic valve is recorded on the right and the tricuspid valve on the left. The RA and LA are visible below the valves.

The apical view. With the transducer placed on the palpable apex, the apical view is obtained. The heart only has two chambers, but routinely the apical views are identified as 4 chamber, 5 chamber and 2 chamber apical view. The 4 chamber view (both atria and ventricles) is obtained with the transducer directed towards the right shoulder; the sectorplane intersects both ventricles in their long axis and is positioned correctly if the RV is as large as possible. This results in a view of both ventricles and both atria with mitral and tricuspid valves (Fig. 2-3, 2-11, 2-12A,B).

With the sectorplane directed more anteriorly, the 5 chamber view shows both ventricles, both atria and the LV outflow tract with the aortic valve and part of the aortic root in one plane.

If the transducer is kept at the apex, but turned 90°, the 2 chamber apical view shows the LV with the outflow tract and the aortic valve with part of the aortic root in one plane.

The subcostal view. If the transducer is placed in the left subcostal region, a few centimeters from the midline, and directed towards the left shoulder, the subcostal view firstly shows part of the liver and behind it the RV and RA. The LV and LA are behind the right heart (Fig. 2-3, 2-13, 2-14). In the adult, echoes from the LV often have a poor quality in this view. The subcostal view is suitable for the evaluation of the right side of the heart and for the inter-atrial septum.

The IVC view. With the transducer in the subcostal region near to the xyphoid, directed almost perpendicular to the abdominal wall and angled slightly to the right side of the patient with the sectorplane in the long axis of the patient, the IVC and hepatic veins are recorded (Fig. 2-4, 2-15, 2-16). The IVC is perpendicular to the transducer, the hepatic veins are parallel to the ultrasound beams. Changes in the diameter of the IVC during respiration can be observed from this view and flow patterns in the hepatic veins can be studied.

The suprasternal view. If the transducer is placed in the suprasternal notch with the sectorplane directed from the right anterior to the left posterior, the suprasternal view is obtained (Fig. 2-3, 2-17, 2-18). In a large percentage of adults a rather good picture can be obtained from a part of the thoracic aorta. Occasionally, a position just above the right clavicle also gives information about the aorta.

References

Feigenbaum H: Echocardiography, 4th ed. Philadelphia, Lea & Febiger, 1986.

Chapter 3. Trans-esophageal echocardiographic examination

Introduction

Today's echocardiographic equipment is capable of providing diagnostic images in most patients. However, the quality of TTE is still limited in some cases. This is due to interference from the chest wall and the lungs. Also, with the apical approach, the far-field areas are visualized sub-optimally as the low-frequency transducers have limited resolution.

TEE is not limited by chest wall interference or thoracic attenuation. Also, the far-field areas from TTE are the near-field areas from TEE. Higher frequency transducers with a better resolution can be used with TEE.

Cardiologists, being used to the more patient friendly TTE technique, may feel intimidated by the esophagoscopic approach and somewhat reluctant to perform it. However, the attitude of the cardiologist to TEE always becomes positive after having done several investigations. Patient acceptance appears to be uniformly good and the cardiologist quickly becomes familiar with the new and better quality cross-sections that can provide much more valuable information.

Proper training in the procedure is important. Initial training can best be provided by a gastroenterologist. With some skill, the introduction and manipulation are readily accomplished. Technicians should not undertake TEE alone.

Indications for TEE

The esophagus is adjacent to the LA and the descending aorta. The high resolution and the shorter distance to the transducer make high quality images of the LA, mitral valve, inter-atrial septum and aortic valve possible. Flow patterns in the heart can be studied in detail. With TTE shielding of the LA by prosthetic valves often prevents evaluation of insufficiencies. TEE with color Doppler provides excellent evaluation of (para)valvular mitral insufficiency. With TEE, the inter-atrial septum is about perpendicular to the transducer and also the detection of a very small ASD is now simple. This is difficult or impossible with TTE. A different and often better evaluation of the aortic valve and RA are possible with TEE; measurements of the size of the LV however are unreliable as the IVS and LVPW are parallel to the ultrasound beams.

A new field of interest in ultrasound diagnosis is the descending aorta. If the scope is rotated anticlockwise, all of the thoracic descending aorta adjacent to the transducer can be visualized. Good information about the presence of dissections and plaques can be obtained. The true and false lumens can be distinguished with color Doppler. The aortic arch and the ascending aorta are not always visible.

The indications for TEE are the following:
- poor TTE imaging
- arterial embolization
- prosthetic valve dysfunction
- aortic dissection
- endocarditis
- cardiac masses
- mitral regurgitation
- evaluation of valve repair during surgery
- LV monitoring during surgery

Information for the patient

TEE is unpleasant for most patients. The idea that something will be introduced into the esophagus can be threatening and some patients expect problems with respiration. In the discussion with the patient this possibility should be denied in advance.

In the conscious patient, TEE is seldom planned far in advance: the indication is usually made after an inconclusive TTE. From patients comments it appears that TEE is better accepted if performed immediately after TTE and the patient had little time to become anxious.

The procedure should be explained by the doctor who does the investigation. During explanation and introduction, the patient should see only the doctor and the assistant since most patients report that the fewer people they see, the better. Also, the presence of more people should be avoided, as the patient then may get the false idea that the procedure is dangerous and unusual. It is also understandable that many patients feel humiliated if they, often without dentures, must retch and feel saliva dripping from the mouth.

The patient is informed that local anesthesia is given with a spray, not with a needle, and that the average examination takes about 10 minutes. Many patients are surprised and somewhat relieved when told of this short duration. We also keep the patient informed about the estimated number of minutes that remain during the examination.

In our experience, premedication is not necessary and may cause serious side effects.

No appreciable bacteremia is associated with simple endoscopic procedures unaccompanied by biopsy. Until now, there is no consensus whether in high risk patients with prosthetic valves prophylaxis should be recommended.

Technique of introduction

Any history of esophageal disease or dysphagia should be elicited. To prevent aspiration the patient should abstain from all oral intake for at least 4 hours.

To avoid damage to the scope, dentures should be removed or a bite guard used. A bite guard however, prevents proper swallowing.

Lidocain spray is given with the patient upright; 6 sprays at the first application, and another 6 sprays the second time. The lidocain is swallowed, so that the upper part of the esophagus is also anaesthesized. Effects occur within 1 minute and persist for 20 minutes.

To avoid aspiration, the patient is in the left decubitus position during introduction and examination. The echocardiographic unit and the assistant are behind the patient. The assistant keeps the part of the scope with the lock controls in his hand. The doctor introduces the scope while facing the patient. The tip of the scope can be lubricated with jelly. The shaft is embedded in a wet gauze and kept in the right hand; a dry scope is inconvenient and more difficult to introduce. The patient's head is comfortably flexed. During introduction with the right hand, the doctor can keep the patient's head flexed with the left hand to avoid introduction into the trachea. The scope is introduced with the tip in the unlocked position and with the transducer facing anteriorly. Any forceful resistance to entering the esophagus should be avoided and introduction is most successful during and immediately after swallowing. This is the difficult part of the procedure: the patient is anxious, retches and has a fear of airway obstruction. Extra secretion of saliva and vomiting reflexes are common. The success of introduction is greater when the procedure is stopped at about 10 cm from the incisors. The patient should be told then to discover that normal breathing is possible. This relieves most patients. Uninterrupted quiet talking to the patient during introduction is reassuring and therefore important.

Further advance is easier during swallowing and should not be painful. A difficult moment may be at a level of about 20 cm from the incisors but by swallowing this point can be passed. If not, just waiting and doing nothing but talking to the patient, even for a few minutes, may relax the patient and the esophagus.

It seems sensible initially to advance the scope as deep as necessary: it is better for the patient to hear that the scope is to be retracted slowly instead of going deeper! Also, further advancement is occasionally difficult or impossible after a 1 or 2 minute inspection of, for example, the aortic valve. This may be caused by contraction of the esophagus. Few patients have problems once the scope is in position. The images are documented on video in order to keep the procedure as short as possible in which case the average examination takes about 10 minutes. The scope should be retracted slowly to prevent unnecessary pain. Because of the local anaesthesia nothing should be taken by mouth for the next 20 minutes.

Complications with TEE are seldom seen: rhythm disturbances have been described incidentally. Abnormalities of the esophagus also can cause complications.

Transducer positions

The position of the esophagus with respect to the heart is illustrated in Fig. 3-1 and 3-2.

Until now, the section planes with TEE have been limited to the horizontal. Presentation of the images has not yet been completely standardized. It is logical to keep the electronics at the same settings as for TTE. Switching the image upside down and/or left to right is only time-consuming. The sections presented here are made without such changes.

At a level of about 40 cm from the incisors, the heart chambers and motion of the heart can be seen. If necessary, the transducer may be slightly rotated to get the heart in the middle of the sector image. With further introduction to 45-50 cm, the liver is readily recognized with part of the ventricles. If anterior rotation of the tip of the scope is possible without any resistance, then it is in the stomach. This permits recording of the apical region of the heart, and, if retracted a few centimeters, a true short axis view of both ventricles is obtained (Fig. 3-3). This section corresponds with section I from Fig. 3-1 and 3-2. Good information about wall thickness, papillary muscles and contraction pattern of the LV can be obtained.

With the scope retracted to a level of about 40 cm, a four chamber view is obtained (Fig. 3-4, 3-5). This section corresponds with section II from Fig. 3-1 and 3-2.

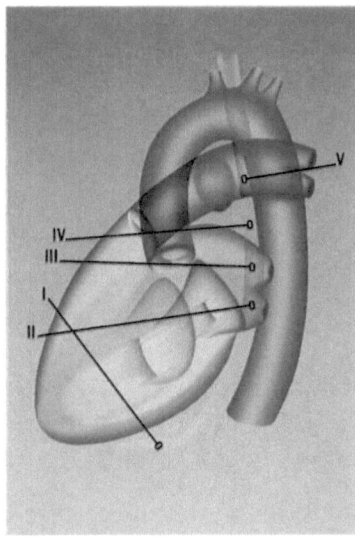

Fig. 3-1. Transparent schematic representation of the heart from the lateral position illustrating the position of the esophagus with respect to the heart. Sections I-V are more or less standardized and refer to Figs. 3-3 to 3-12.

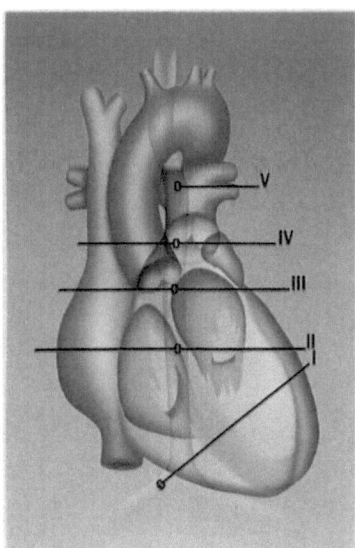

Fig. 3-2. Transparant schematic representation of the heart in the antero-posterior direction, illustrating the position of the esophagus with respect to the heart.

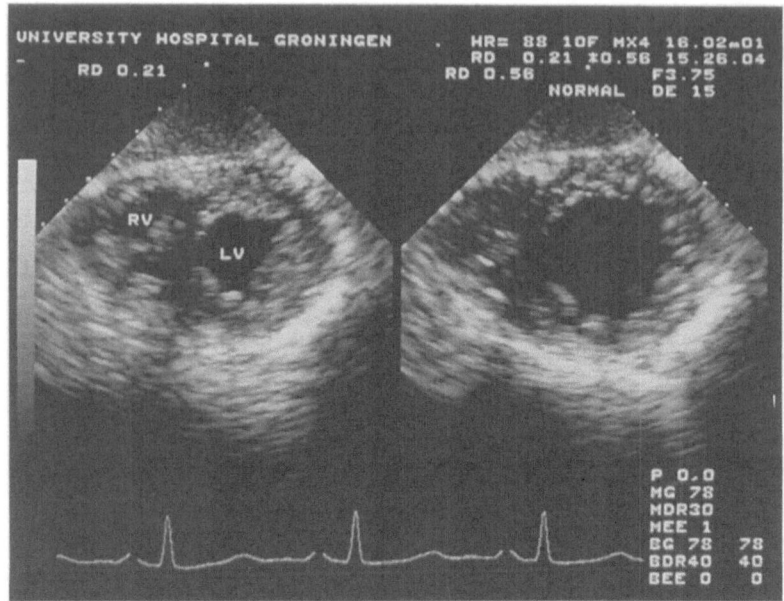

Fig. 3-3. Trans-gastric short axis view of the ventricles during systole (left) and diastole.

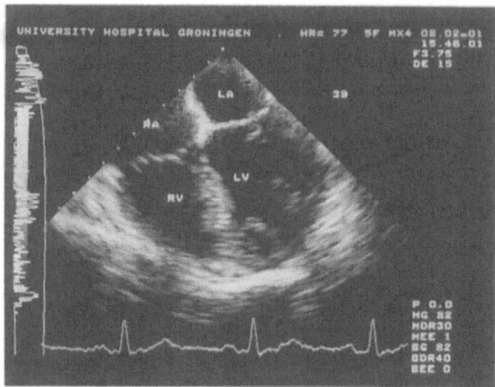

Fig. 3-4. Mid-systolic frame of a four chamber view of the heart, obtained with TEE. The LA is adjacent to the esophagus. The LV with part of the papillary muscles is visible below the closed mitral valve.

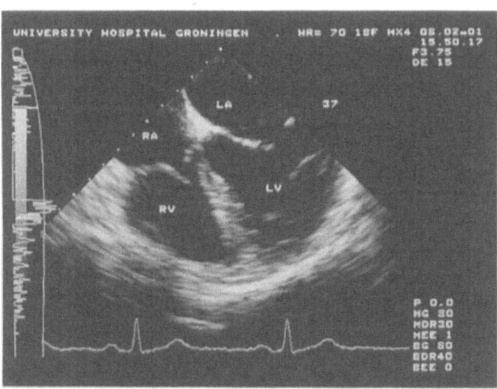

Fig. 3-5. Diastolic frame of a four chamber view of the heart from the same position as in Fig. 3-4.

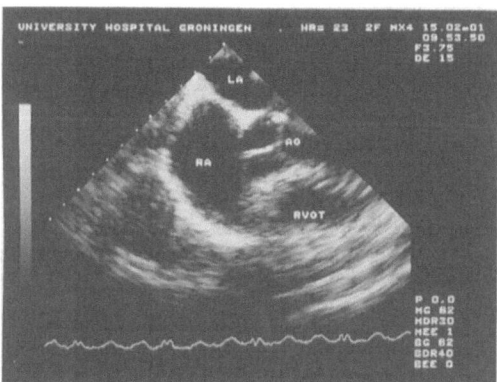

Fig. 3-6. Section through the aortic valve (AO), LA, RA and RV outflow tract (RVOT). Note that the aortic valve ring is not 'closed' as the plane through the ring has an angle with respect to the section plane.

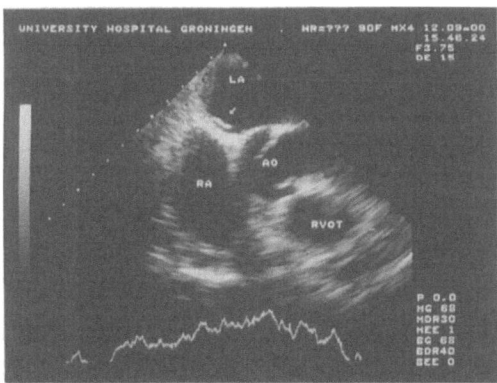

Fig. 3-7. Systolic frame at the level of the aortic valve (AO) and RV outflow tract (RVOT). Between LA and RA the valvula of the fossa ovalis is visible (arrow).

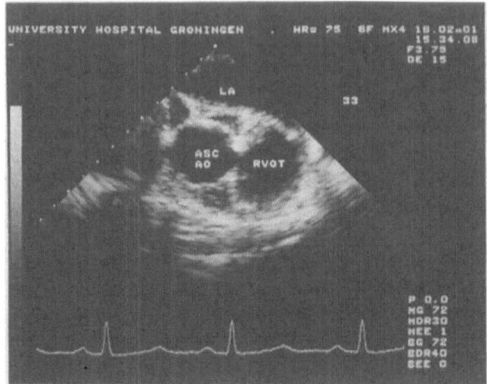

Fig. 3-8. Transverse section through the ascending aorta (ASC AO) just above the aortic valve. The triangular area on the left of the picture is the superior vena cava. The smaller triangular area between the LA and the ascending aorta and RVOT is not a vessel but the transverse sinus, an extension of the pericardial sac.

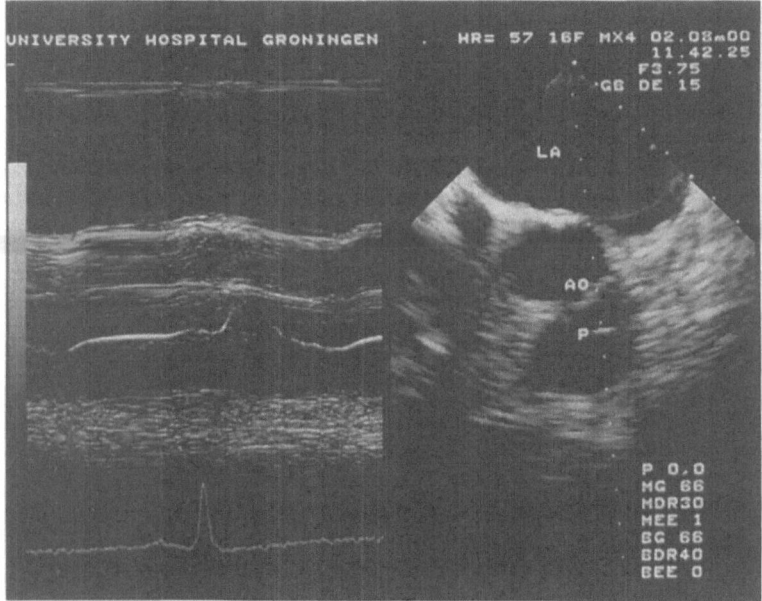

Fig. 3-9. This section through the LA and the ascending aorta (AO) shows part of the pulmonic valve (P). On the M-mode recording a mirror image of the valve is seen if compared with the well-known recording from TTE.

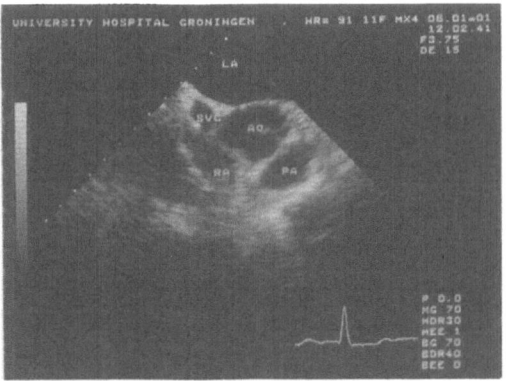

Fig. 3-10. Section through the aorta (AO) and the pulmonary artery (PA). Between LA and RA the superior vena cava (SVC) is visible as a small, almost circular structure.

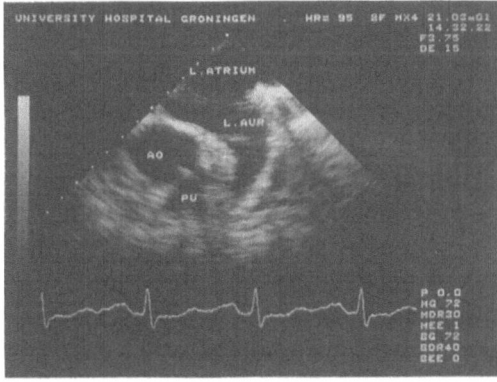

Fig. 3-11. The LA with the left auricle (L.AUR) in front of the ascending aorta (AO) and the pulmonic valve (PV).

The four chamber TEE view cannot be compared with that obtained with TTE; Fig. 3-2 shows that the long axis of the LV makes an angle with respect to the section plane. In fact, the distal LV wall is not the apex, but part of the anterior wall. Measurement of the LV long axis is not reliable. The position of the endocardium of the LV is not always clear as there is hardly any angle between the ultrasound beams and the endocardium. Consequently, endocardial definition is impaired. This section is suitable for the evaluation of the mitral apparatus, the LV outflow tract, the inter-atrial septum with its central thinned fossa ovalis membrane, the RA and the tricuspid valve.

At a level of about 30-35 cm a section is obtained through the aortic valve with both atria and the RV outflow tract (Fig. 3-6). This section corresponds

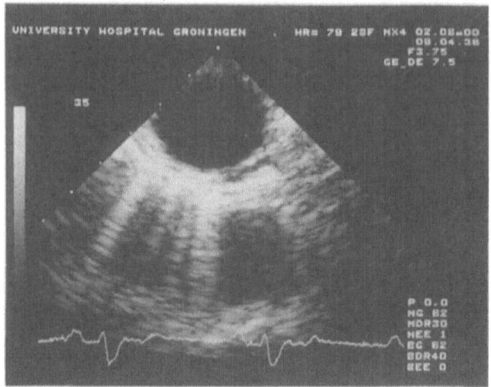

Fig. 3-12. Transverse section through the circular shaped descending aorta with the left pulmonary artery at a level of 35 cm. Note a different scale from that of the other figures.

with section III from Fig. 3-1 and 3-2.

The origin of both coronary arteries can often be seen. A perfect cross section through the aortic valve ring with the three cusps is usually not obtained as the plane of the aortic valve ring has an angle with respect to the horizontal plane. Also at this level, the inter-atrial septum is usually hit perpendicular to the beam. The valvula of the fossa ovalis can often be recorded (Fig. 3-7).

Above the aortic valve ring the circular shaped aortic root is recorded with the RV outflow tract more posterior (Fig. 3-8).

The upper portion of the ascending aorta cannot be visualized as the trachea interferes.

For recording the pulmonic valve with TEE, the direction of the ultrasound beam is often almost as poor as with the TTE approach. Also, poorly conducting mediastinal tissue often interferes as the esophagus is usually no longer in contact with the heart at this level (Fig. 3-1 and 3-2, section IV). An M-mode recording of the the pulmonic valve with TEE is sometimes possible and shows a mirror image of the well known recording with TTE (Fig. 3-9). The superior vena cava is usually also most visible at this level (Fig. 3-10).

Rotating the scope somewhat anti-clockwise permits recording of the left auricle (Fig. 3-11).

Rotating the scope 90-120° anticlockwise permits visualization of a horizontal section through the descending aorta (Fig. 3-12). This section corresponds with section V from Fig. 3-1 and 3-2.

For aortic dissection good images are obtained with TEE. Intermittently, the scope can be rotated from the heart to the aorta and back at various levels. Also, the whole descending aorta can be visualized continuously. As the relationship between the esophagus and the aorta changes at various levels, less anti-clockwise rotation will be necessary if the transducer is positioned more cranially.

The upper part of the descending aorta can be visualized by rotating the scope anti-clockwise. Most of the transverse aortic arch and part of the ascending aorta can usually be seen.

The esophagoscope

The transducer is incorporated into the flexible tip of a gastroscope which is calibrated for depth. This is the most vulnerable part of the scope. Most scopes become defective because of direct mechanical damage to the transducer. Less often a bite from a patient is the cause. Special care should be taken that the tip of the scope is safe during storage. A construction is recommended in which the shaft hangs in a transparent tube.

After each use, the scope should be washed and cleaned and hung in a tube filled with glutaraldehyde solution (Cidex) for at least 15 minutes. After this, the glutaral should be removed carefully and the scope washed before the next use. If the scope is not being used, it should be stored dry in order not to damage the transducer elements.

References

Schlüter M, Langenstein BA, Polster J, Kremer P, Souquet J, Engel S, Hanrath P: Transoesophageal cross-section echocardiography with a phased array transducer system. Technique and initial clinical results. Br Heart J 48:67, 1982.

Seward JB, Khandheria BK, Oh JK, Abel MD, Hughes RW, Edwards WD, Nichols BA, Freeman WK, Tajik AJ: Trans-esophageal echocardiography: technique, anatomic correlations, implementation, and clinical applications. Mayo Clin Proc 63:649, 1988.

Erbel R, Borner N, Steller D, Brunier J, Thelen M, Pfeiffer C, Mohr-Kahaly S, Iversen S, Oelert H, Meyer J: Detection of aortic dissection by trans-esophageal echocardiography. Br Heart J 58(1):45, 1987.

Dahm M, Iversen S, Schmid FX, Drexler M, Erbel R, Oelert H: Intraoperative evaluation of reconstruction of the atrioventricular valves by transesophageal echocardiography. Thorac Cardiovasc Surg 35 (2) 140, 1987.

Erbel R, Rohmann S, Drexler M, Mohr-Kahaly S, Gerharz CD, Iversen S, Oelert H, Meyer J: Improved diagnostic value of echocardiography in patients with infective endocarditis by transesophageal approach. A prospective study. Eur Heart J 9(1):43, 1988.

Seward JB, Tajik AJ, DiMagno EP: Esophageal phased-array sector echocardiography: an anatomic study. In: Hanrath P, Bleifeld W, Souquet J eds. Cardiovascular Diagnosis by ultrasound. The Hague:Martinus Nijhoff:270, 1982.

De Bruijn NP, Clements FM: Transesophageal echocardiography. Dordrecht, Martinus Nijhoff Publishing, 1987.

Chapter 4. Contrast echocardiography

Spontaneous contrast can be seen in the heart if flow velocities are very low such as in the LA in mitral stenosis (Fig. 4-1, 4-2) and in the LV in dilating cardiomyopathy. Also with TEE from prosthetic valves, spontaneous contrast can be found. If good quality pictures can be made, spontaneaous contrast can also be found in a normal IVC and in normal liver veins.

If saline, glucose, dextrose or other such solutions are injected into a peripheral vein or into the heart, a cloud of echoes will be recorded on the echocardiogram (Fig. 4-3).

In the past, contrast echocardiography has been used for identification of endocardium, the detection of shunts, flow patterns, valve insufficiencies etc. and for the evaluation of myocardial perfusion. An example of the use of contrast echocardiography in the diagnosis of tricuspid regurgitation is presented in Fig. 4-4. In case of tricuspid insufficiency, 'contrast' can also be found in the IVC and hepatic veins, if injected in the brachial vein (Fig. 4-5).

With the advent of Doppler echocardiography, especially color flow imaging, contrast echocardiography has been superseded. Valve insufficiencies can now be detected easily with Doppler. However, not every hospital has a color Doppler system or a TEE system.

For the diagnosis of ASD, a case remains for contrast echocardiography. The detection of an ASD in the adult can be difficult with echocardiography alone, but also with Doppler echocardiography, or even color Doppler. If 10 cc glucose 5% is injected forcefully into a peripheral vein, a cloud of echoes will first appear in the RA and then in the RV. Prior to injection the syringe can be shaken. This often results in an increased intensity of echoes. As many ASD's also have a small right-to-left shunt, part of the 'contrast' may pass through the inter-atrial septum and appear in the LA. If, in the presence of an ASD, an M-mode recording is made from the LA during injection, some 'contrast' will be seen there before the RV becomes opaque. This is still a good and reliable method for the detection of an ASD.

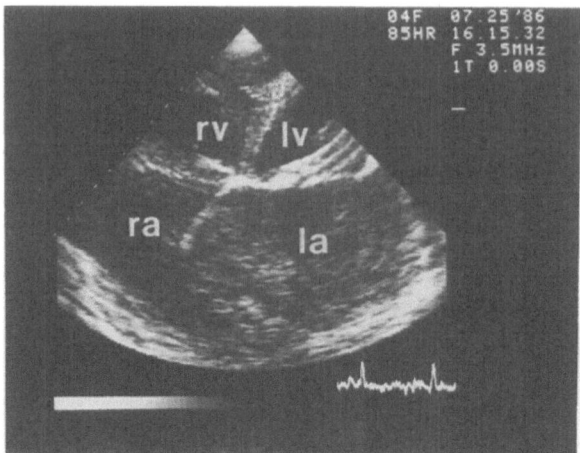

Fig. 4-1. Apical view in mitral stenosis. The LV is small. The LA is the largest compartment and is filled with clouds of echoes: spontaneous contrast is visible because the flow velocities in the LA are very low. In the moving picture these echoes whirl slowly around.

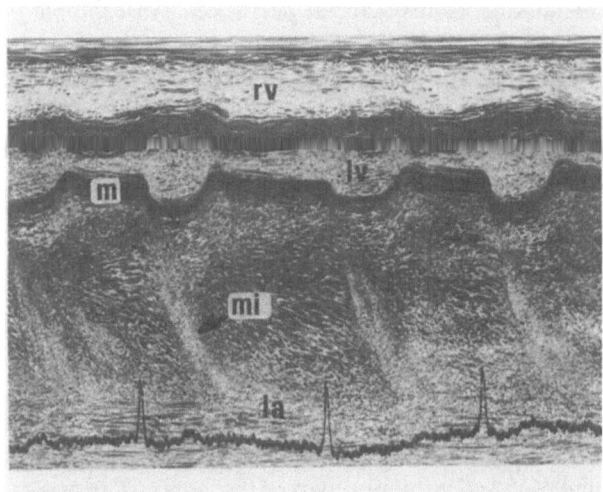

Fig. 4-2. Long axis M-mode recording. The LV is small, the mitral valve (m) is stenotic. The LA is greatly enlarged and filled with spontaneous contrast. The opacity in the contrast during systole is caused by concomittant mitral insufficiency (mi).

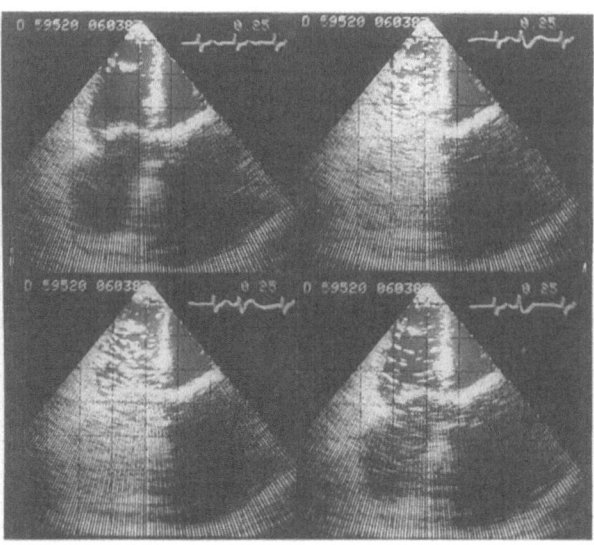

Fig. 4-3. Apical view before (upper left) and after injection of 10 cc glucose 5% in the brachial vein. The 'contrast' fills the right side of the heart immediately (upper right, lower left) and tends to disappear in the normal heart after 12-16 heartbeats (lower right).

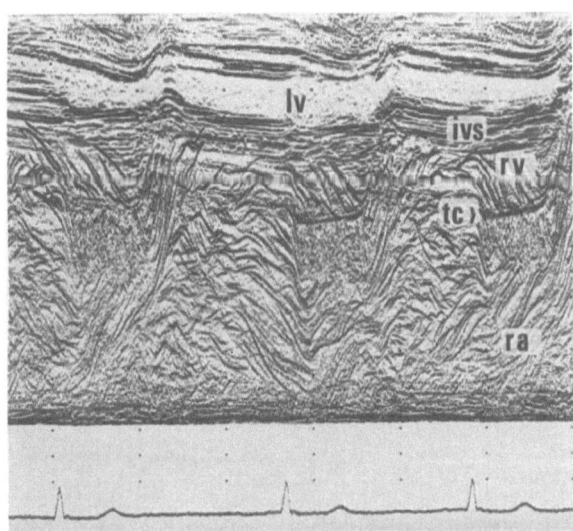

Fig. 4-4. Apical M-mode recording through LV, IVS and RV to RA. Glucose has been injected in the brachial vein and is visible in the right heart. During systole the contrast passes the tricuspid closure line (tc) with a high velocity, indicating tricuspid insufficiency.

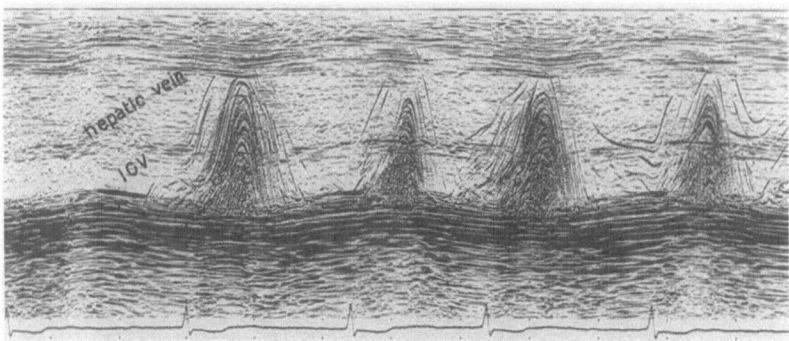

Fig. 4-5. IVC view with hepatic vein after injection of glucose 5% in the brachial vein. The presence of contrast in both veins proves tricuspid insufficiency.

References

Seward JB, Tajik AJ, Spangler JG, Ritter DG: Echocardiographic contrast studies: Intitial experience. Mayo Clin Proc 50:163, 1975.

Shub C, Tajik AJ, Hagler DJ, Ritter DG: Peripheral venous contrast echocardiography. Am J Cardiol 39:202, 1977.

Bommer WJ, Shah PM, Allen H, Meltzer R, Kisslo J: The safety of contrast echocardiography: Report of the Committee on Contrast Echocardiography for the American Society of Echocardiography. J Am Coll Cardiol 3:6, 1984.

Tei C, Sakamaki T, Shah PM, Meerbaum S, Shimoura K, Kondo S, Crday E: Myocardial contrast echocardiography: A reproducible technique of myocardial opacification for identifying regional perfusion deficits. Circulation 67:585, 1983.

Chapter 5. Phonocardiography and pulse recording

Introduction

Phonocardiography is used to identify murmurs and heart sounds with their relative loudness. Recordings of motion patterns of the heart, vessels and liver are useful for the identification and the detection of the severity of heart diseases.

The role of phonocardiography and pulse recording has lost some of its importance since the advent of echocardiography and Doppler. Before echocardiography, non-invasive diagnosis of heart disease and its severity was made with only the patients history, physical examination and auscultation, electrocardiography and chest X-ray, phonocardiography and pulse recording. However, auscultation and echocardiography did not replace phonocardiography. Phonocardiography on the other hand, never replaced auscultation: due to technical limitations the technique occasionally fails to detect audible sounds and murmurs and cannot replace the human ear. Timing of events however, may be difficult with auscultation. For this, phonocardiography and pulse recordings are excellent. Also, the technique is very useful for understanding the events in the heart.

In a non-invasive laboratory the combination of phonocardiography and echo-Doppler is useful for the identification of sounds and murmurs and for the diagnosis and estimation of the severity of heart diseases. For this, phonocardiography and pulse recordings can be used alone or as reference signals on the echocardiographic M-mode recording. For nearly every echocardiograph both are optional, but should be standard.

It is impossible to discuss all aspects of phonocardiography in one Chapter and it is also beyond the scope of this book. Only a few recordings from which measurements can be made will be discussed. Many calculations and several 'normal values' are used; only the values used in the authors institution are presented.

For the calculation of the isovolumic contraction- and relaxation times (IVCT, IVRT) of the ventricles, the moments of closure and opening of cardiac valves can be recorded with high-speed dual M-mode echocardiography. Often such recordings cannot be obtained or are not satisfactory, in which case, a simultanous recording of the aortic or pulmonic closure sound on the M-mode recording can be helpful.

The LV ejection time (LVET) can be important for the estimation of various left sided heart diseases such as aortic stenosis. It is not always possible to obtain the pressure difference across a stenotic aortic valve with CW Doppler. The LVET, then, can be helpful for the estimation of the severity, in combination with a recording of the systolic murmur.

The LVET can be calculated from a high-speed M-mode recording from the aortic valve. For most normal aortic valves recording of the exact moments of opening and closure is successful, but in case of e.g. a calcified aortic stenosis it can be very difficult or impossible. The LVET can then be calculated from the carotid pulse recording; it can give a good indication for the severity of aortic stenosis. Many other factors however, influence the duration of the LVET.

The apexcardiogram can provide good information about the LV end-diastolic pressure by calculating the a-wave. Jugular and liver pulse recordings are helpful in the diagnosis and especially the severity of tricuspid regurgitation.

Phonocardiogram

For phonocardiographic reference signals on the echocardiogram a poor-quality microphone is usually supplied; in most cases it should be replaced by a better quality one. The microphone can be attached to the chest. It can also be held by hand in which case a second examiner may be needed. The localization of the microphone on the chest depends on the problem being investigated and on the transducer position. Firstly, the transducer position should be known. The best position for the microphone can be found with auscultation.

With most equipments a choice can be made between high, medium and low frequency recordings. Usually the best choice for recording a heart sound is the medium frequency; high frequencies often have a poor technical quality and with low frequencies the exact moment at which a sound starts is difficult to determine. For calculations, recordings should be made at a speed of 100 mm/sec.

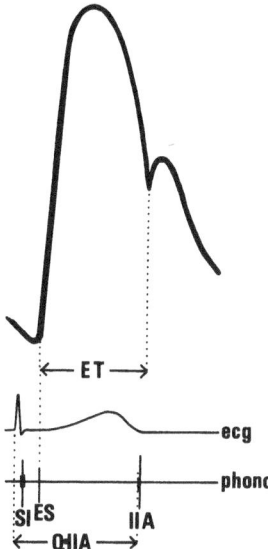

Fig. 5-1. A schematic carotid pulse recording using the method of calculation of ejection time (ET) and electromechanical interval (Q-IIA). S1 = first heart sound, ES = aortic ejection sound, IIA = aortic closure sound.

Pulse recordings

Carotid pulse recording and systolic time intervals

If the pick up device for pulse recording is placed on the carotid artery in the mid-neck region, the carotid pulse recording is obtained. The filling of the carotid artery starts with a positive deflection and ends with the incisura. The incisura is preceded by the aortic closure sound and helps to differentiate it from the pulmonic closure sound. The initial rapid ascent of the carotid pulse recording identifies an aortic ejection sound that may be present very close to this moment.

The ejection time is the time between the initial rapid ascent and the incisura (Fig. 5-1). Factors that lengthen the ejection time are, for example, aortic stenosis, aortic insufficiency, hypertension and coarctation. Factors that shorten the ejection time are, for example, mitral insufficiency, a poor LV function and impaired LV filling as in mitral stenosis or hypovolemia.

As the ejection time also depends on heart rate and sex, it has to be corrected for both. The corrected ejection time is called the ejection time index (ETI) (Table 1).

The total duration of the LV systole (or the electromechanical interval) is the time between the onset of the ECG and the aortic closure sound, the

Q-IIA interval. This interval also depends on heart rate and sex and has to be corrected for both. This results in the Q-IIAc.

If the ejection time is subtracted from the Q-IIA, the pre-ejection period (PEP) is obtained. This is an indirect measurement of the isovolumic contraction period. The PEP value should be corrected for the heart rate to obtain the PEPc.

The ratio PEP/LVET is a useful index for the prediction of cardiac output and good correlations have been found with fractional shortening and ejection fraction of the LV.

Note: if the PEP/ET is used for estimating the 'quality' of the LV, it is only valuable if there are no significant valve abnormalities (see factors, influencing the ejection time)

Apexcardiogram

If the pick up device for pulse recording is placed at the palpable apex of the heart, the apexcardiogram (ACG) can be recorded. The normal ACG has a positive deflection during ventricular systole (Fig. 5-2).

The deflection starts at the R of a normal QRS complex and reaches its maximum at point E in early systole; during the second half of systole a plateau is usually reached. A sustained rise after point E however, can also be found in normal individuals. Shortly before the aortic closure sound a sharp downward motion is recorded that ends at point O, the moment that the mitral valve has just been opened. This is followed by a steep rise, the rapid filling (rf) period

Table 1. Calculation of the corrected values of the systolic time intervals according to Weissler. Q-IIA = electromechanical interval: time between Q of ECG and aortic closure sound. Q-IIAc = Q-IIA, corrected for heart rate and sex. LVET = LV ejection time: time between upstroke of the carotid pulse recording and the carotid incisura. ETI = ejection time index: the LVET corrected for heart rate and sex. PEP = pre-ejection period. PEPc = PEP, corrected for heart rate. HR = heart rate. n = normal values with standard deviation.

Systolic time intervals with normal values

♂	Q-IIAc	$= Q\text{-IIA} + 2.1 \times HR$	$n = 546 \pm 14$ ms
♀	Q-IIAc	$= Q\text{-IIA} + 2.0 \times HR$	$n = 549 \pm 14$ ms
♂	ETI	$= LVET + 1.7 \times HR$	$n = 413 \pm 10$ ms
♀	ETI	$= LVET + 1.6 \times HR$	$n = 418 \pm 10$ ms
	PEP	$= Q\text{-IIAc} - LVET$	
♂	PEPc	$= PEP + 0.4 \times HR$	$n = 131 \pm 13$ ms
♀	PEPc	$= PEP + 0.4 \times HR$	$n = 133 \pm 11$ ms
	PEP/LVET:		$n = 0.345 \pm 0.035$

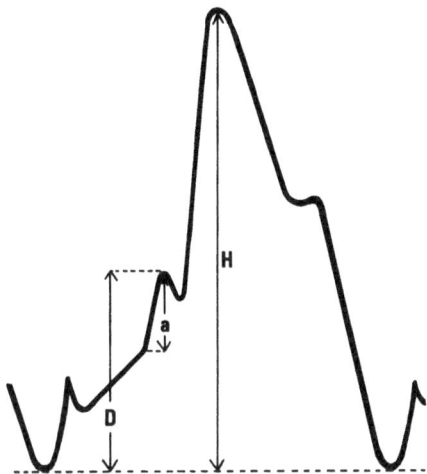

Fig. 5-2. A schematic apexcardiogram with the method of calculation of the a/H and a/D ratio. D = total diastolic deflection, a = deflection caused by atrial contraction, H = total deflection of the apexcardiogram.

that ends with the rf point. If there is a third heart sound, it coincides with this point. Then, the slow filling phase is recorded, that ends in a small positive deflection, the a-wave: an outward motion of the LV, caused by the LA contraction. A possible fourth heart sound coincides with the top of the a-wave.

To some extent, the magnitude of the a-wave reflects the end-diastolic pressure of the LV (LVEDP). Thus, the a-wave is helpful in assessing the severity of various heart diseases. Measurement of the a-wave is made as a percentage of the total deflection (H) of the ACG, the a/H ratio. The normal a/H ratio is less than 12%. The number of percentages of the a/H ratio is often the same as the number of mm Hg of the LVEDP. The size of the a-wave can also be expressed as a percentage of the total diastolic deflection (D), the a/D ratio. This ratio should be less than 36%.

Liver pulse recording

With the pick up device in the right subcostal zone as lateral as possible, pulsations of the liver can be recorded. The recording can be used to estimate the severity of tricuspid insufficiency.

The liver pulse recording resembles the jugular venous pulse recording. Because of damping by the liver itself, all events occur a short time later and the deflections are not as sharply marked as with the jugular pulse. However, most patients with tricuspid insufficiency have a preferential flow towards the IVC en sometimes reflections of tricuspid insufficiency are better evaluated

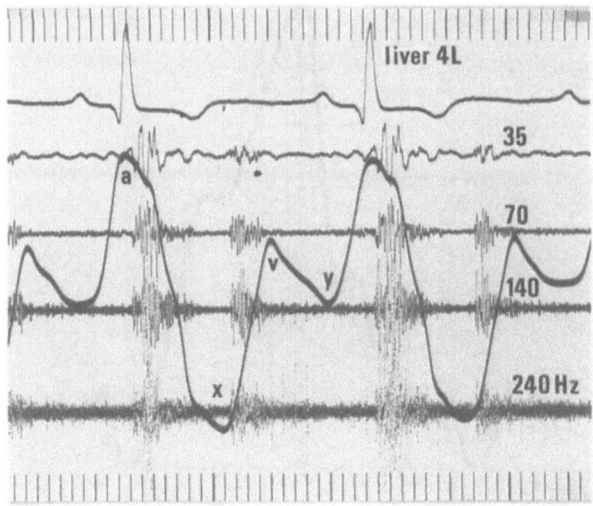

Fig. 5-3. Normal liver pulse recording with simultaneous recording of heart sounds and murmurs on the 4th rib on the left side of the sternum. Cut-of frequencies of the phonocardiogram are at 35, 70, 140 and 240 Hz. See text for further explanation. The pattern of the liver pulse recording is similar to that of the jugular pulse recording, but somewhat delayed and dampened.

from the liver pulse recording (Fig. 5-3).

During atrial systole a positive deflection, the a-wave, shows the absence of valves between the RA and the IVC: the RA not only pumps blood into the the RV, but also into the liver. This deflection is followed by a negative deflection during RV systole, the x-descent, caused by atrial relaxation and a downward motion of the tricuspid ring. The tracing then rises again, representing filling of the RA, and ends in the v-wave. This is followed by the y-descent that starts after opening of the tricuspid valves. Normally, the a-wave is the highest and the x-descent the lowest point of the tracing.

In case of tricuspid insufficiency, the x-descent is filled up by the regurgiting blood. The more severe the tricuspid insufficiency is, the earlier the filling starts, resulting in a positive s-wave. In very severe tricuspid insufficiency the deflection of the tracing is only positive during RV systole.

References

Weissler AM, Harris WS, Schoenfeld CD: Bedside technics for the evaluation of ventricular function in man. Am J Cardiol 23:577, 1969.

Weissler AM, Harris WS, Schoenfeld CD: Systolic time intervals in heart failure in man. Circulation XXXVII No 2:149, 1968.

Tavel ME: Clinical Phonocardiography and external pulse recording. 4th ed. Chicago, Year book medical publishers, 1985.

Chapter 6. Principles of doppler

Introduction

As in echo, man was not the first to use the principle of Doppler for the estimation of velocities. The dolphin can not only estimate distances but it is also capable of detecting its own velocity with respect to motionless structures and also the difference in velocity between itself and fishes.

If sound waves are compressed, a higher frequency will be obtained; if they are stretched, the frequency will be lower. From audible sound this Doppler principle is experienced in daily life from trains, motor cars, airplanes etc. (Fig. 6-1). If they come towards the observer, a higher pitched sound will be heard than that produced by the object. If they go away from the observer, a lower pitched sound will be heard.

It is not important if the sound producing object or the observer is moving: they just have to move in relation to each other to obtain the Doppler effect. If a transducer produces ultrasound of a certain frequency which is reflected by an object moving towards the transducer, the echoes will have a higher frequency than the produced ultrasound. The difference between the frequencies of the emitted and the reflected ultrasound is called the Doppler shift. The motion of an object towards the transducer causes a positive Doppler shift, away from the transducer a negative Doppler shift. A higher velocity of the object will result in a greater Doppler shift.

The Doppler examination can be performed with the continuous wave Doppler (CW) or with the pulsed Doppler (PD) technique.

Continuous wave Doppler

With CW, one crystal transmits ultrasound continuously, and (an)other crystal (s) receive(s) (Fig. 6-2). The transmitted ultrasound is represented by a dotted

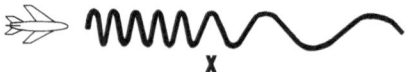

Fig. 6-1. Demonstration of the Doppler effect. If an airplane goes in the direction of an observer (X), the sound waves produced by the airplane are compressed and the observer will hear a higher pitched sound than that, produced by the airplane. If it moves away from the observer, a lower pitched sound will be heard, caused by stretching of the sound waves. The shift in frequency between the sound that was really produced and the sound that is heard is called the Doppler shift.

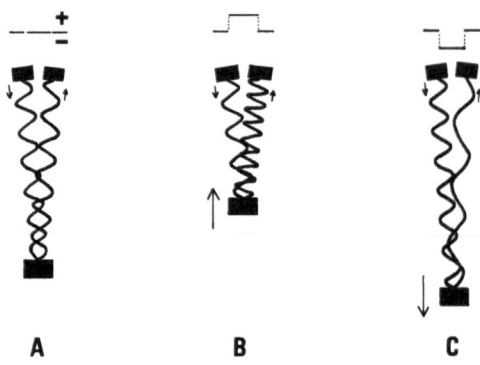

Fig. 6-2. The principle of CW Doppler. At A the left sided crystal emits sound of a specific frequency that reflects against an immobile object: the same frequency is found in the echoes and the Doppler shift is zero. At B the object moves towards the transducer and causes compression of the sound: the Doppler shift is positive and a positive deflection is recorded. At C the object moves away from the transducer, resulting in a negative Doppler shift.

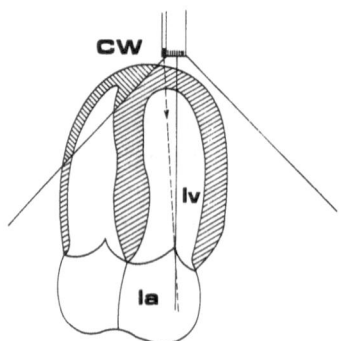

Fig. 6-3. Schematic representation of the heart from the apical view. The transducer continuously emits the ultrasound for Doppler by a separate crystal (dotted line) and receives the signal along the straight line.

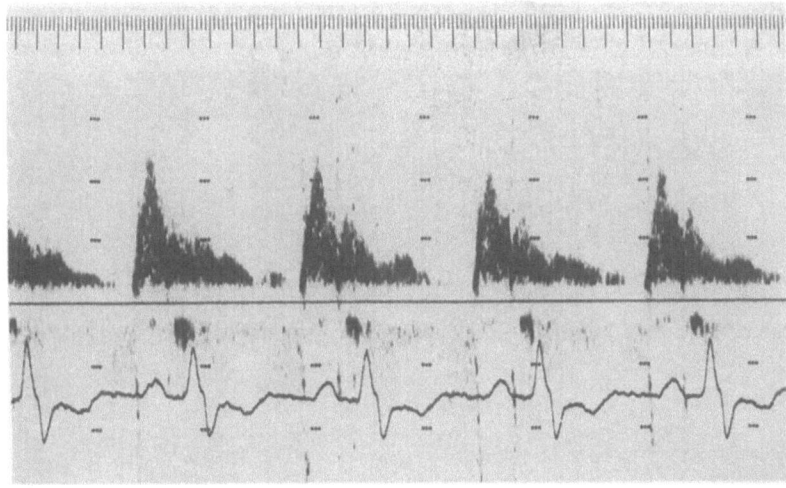

Fig. 6-4. CW Doppler signal of the mitral valve from the apical position of a patient with a dilated cardiomyopathy. The flow is directed towards the transducer and the signal will be positive during diastole. However, the Doppler signal does not end at the R of the ECG when the LV starts to contract. Almost throughout systole the signal remains positive, still indicating a flow towards the transducer with a closed mitral valve. This systolic signal is caused by the flow that still goes in the direction of the apex and is also picked up by the CW system, as this system can hardly measure in depth.

line, the direction from which the signal is received is represented by a straight line. In Fig. 6-2 both lines cross at the level of the mitral valve, resulting in some preference for the measurement in that area; however, echoes from the whole depth will be recorded.

Accordingly, it is hardly possible to determine from which depth along the Doppler sound beam a particular velocity was obtained: there is hardly any orientation in depth. In practice this limitation is not confusing as it is nearly always known from the echocardiogram where a maximal velocity can be expected along the Doppler sound beam. Fig. 6-4 shows an example of a CW signal obtained from the LV from the apical position.

All velocities along the line of the Doppler sound beam are recorded: during systole a flow velocity is recorded into the direction of the transducer. It was caused by the still existing inflow in an enlarged LV with a closed mitral valve (Fig. 6-5).

Since with CW, ultrasound is emitted continuously, very high velocities can be detected, which is an advantage of CW.

In adult TTE Doppler-echocardiography CW is often used in combination with PD.

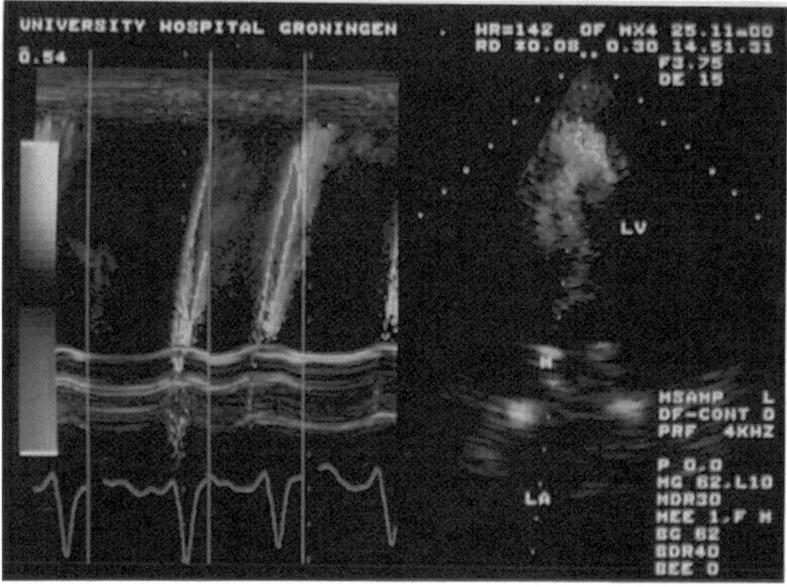

Fig. 6-5. Sector from the apex, frozen during early systole. The prosthetic mitral valve is closed already, but a red color, especially in the apical region still indicates a flow towards the transducer. This explains Fig. 6-3 where during systole a positive Doppler shift still is found. The low velocity of the filling of the LV is visible from the M-mode recording.

Pulsed Doppler

The distance from the transducer is expressed by the time that is needed for ultrasound to be transmitted and reflected. With Doppler, as in echocardio-graphy, distances can only be measured with a pulsed system. With PD, ultrasound pulses of a short duration, 'sound packets', are emitted (Fig. 6-6).

After transmission the echoes are sampled with a specific time delay. This time delay enables the determination of a particular depth. So, accurate determinination of sample positions with a good orientation in depth is an advantage of PD (Fig. 6-7).

A limitation of PD is that measurements of high velocities at a given depth are limited by the frequency of the transducer and the number of pulses per second (pulse repetition frequency = PRF). A high PRF and a low frequency transducer are needed to detect high velocities. If the velocity is too high for a given PRF and transducer frequency, the signal will show aliasing.

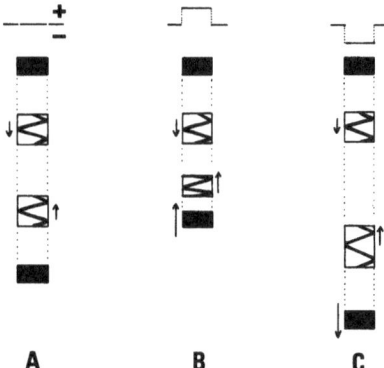

Fig. 6-6. The principle of PD Doppler. At A the transducer emits a sound package towards an immobile object. The returning sound package will have the same frequency: the Doppler shift is zero, there is no deflection on the recording. At B the object moves towards the transducer and causes a higher frequency within the sound package: the Doppler shift is positive with a positive deflection from the baseline. At C the object moves away from the transducer, causing a negative Doppler shift.

Aliasing

Aliasing is inherent to PD in case of high velocities. The phenomenon of aliasing is well known in daily life. If a propeller or a spoked wheel slowly starts to rotate clockwise, a clockwise rotation will be observed indeed. The faster the rotation is, the faster the clockwise rotation will be seen, until the moment that it seems to slow down. While the rotation is actually accelerating, the visible rotation seems to stop. With a further increase in velocity it seems to rotate anticlockwise. This apparent reverse motion may be called aliasing. Rotating faster and faster, the wheel seems to stop again, then seems to rotate clockwise again etc.

A direction will be observed correctly or incorrectly depending on velocity and observation intervals. High velocities may be recorded as going in the opposite direction. A high flow velocity going towards the transducer may be recorded as going away from the transducer.

Angle

The Doppler shift is measured correctly if the motion of an object is exactly towards or away from the transducer. The magnitude of the Doppler shift then only depends on the velocity of the object. However, if an object moves perpendicularly to the transducer a Doppler shift will not be detected. So, the

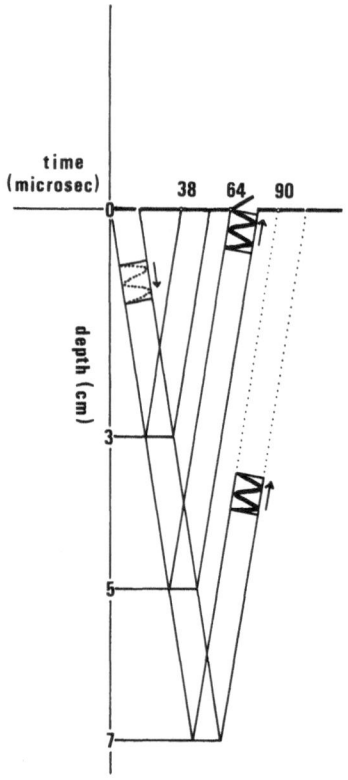

Fig. 6-7. Schematic representation of the method used to obtain signals from a certain distance from the transducer. At time 0 a sound package is emitted. If the area of interest should be at 5 cm from the transducer, the time, needed for ultrasound to travel 2x5 cm is 64 microsec. If the transducer is only 'open' a few microseconds after 64 ms, only the ultrasound waves from a distance of 5 cm will be received. Signals that arrive earlier (for example from 3 cm distance) meet a 'closed' receiver and are not recorded. The signal returning from a depth of 7 cm will return to the transducer later and also finds the receiver 'closed'.

magnitude of the Doppler shift also depends on the angle between the direction of the ultrasound beam and the direction of the flow. The larger the angle, the more the velocity is under-estimated.

The Doppler shift can be calculated using the following equation:

$$f_d = 2f_0 \frac{v . \cos \alpha}{c} \qquad \text{or} \qquad v = \frac{c . f_d}{2f_0 . \cos \alpha}$$

f_d = Doppler shift

f_0 = transmitted ultrasonic frequency

v = velocity of the object

α = angle ultrasound beam / direction of flow

c = velocity of ultrasound in blood (1560 m/s)

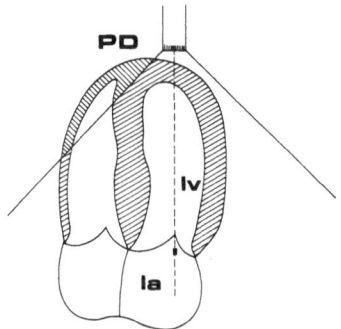

Fig. 6-8. Schematic representation of the heart from the apical view. The transducer emits sound packages along the interrupted line. The position on the line (the sample position) can be changed to obtain a certain depth, in the example just below the mitral leaflets.

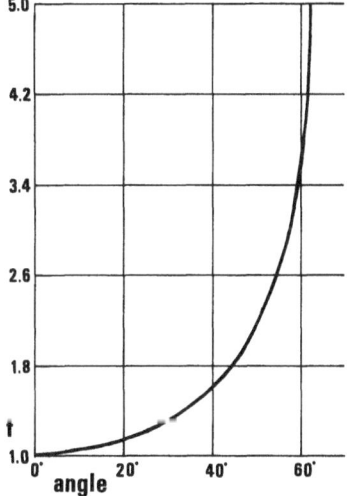

Fig. 6-9. The relationship between the magnitude of the angle between the direction of the ultrasound beam and the direction of the flow, and the factor (f) with which the measured velocity has to be multiplied to obtain the correct velocity.

As a consequence of the cosine function, the factor with which the velocity must be multiplied is not linear (Fig. 6-9): the multiplication factor is unimportant for small angles, and very large for large angles. At an angle of about 60°, a small error in the calculation of the angle causes a large error in the calculation of the flow velocity.

The effect of an angle on the presence or intensity of colors is easy to understand in the aorta. However, this effect should not be forgotten when flow velocities in the ventricles or atria are evaluated.

54

Measurement of pressure differences

If blood flow velocities are known across valves or defects, the difference between pressures on both sides can be measured. To this, the Bernoulli equation is simplified to $p = 4v^2$:

Bernoulli equation

$$p_1 - p_2 = \tfrac{1}{2}\rho(v_2^2 - v_1^2) + \rho\int_1^2 \frac{dv}{dt}\,ds + R(v)$$

$$p = 4v^2$$

Color Doppler

With PD the exact location of a sample is known. This sample position is visualized in the sector image. The magnitude of the Doppler shift, found at that sample position can also be projected on the sector image. Such a Doppler shift at a specific place can be coded with a color. Rather illogically, the agreement has been made that a positive Doppler shift (towards the transducer) is coded red and a negative shift is coded blue. A small Doppler shift is projected as a dark color, a large shift as a bright color.

If numerous samples are taken at almost the same time, numerous color 'dots' fill up the picture there, where Doppler shifts could be detected. It should be kept in mind that a color area, visualized with this method, does not necessarily represent correct flow velocities, but flow velocities as detected from that specific transducer position (angle).

As color Doppler is PD, the specific advantage (orientation in depth) and limitation (aliasing) of PD are also found in color Doppler. Aliasing of color Doppler results in the opposite color (opposite direction).

For the explanation of color Doppler with advantages and limitations the signals from the thoracic aorta from the suprasternal position can be used. The direction of flow is known there as are velocities and velocity profiles (Fig. 6-10 and 6-11).

In the ascending aorta the direction of the flow in Fig. 6-10 is towards the transducer but not exactly in line with the direction of the ultrasound beams. The angle between both causes under-estimation of the velocity. However, the angle for this region is only small and under-estimation will not be important. In the horizontal part of the aorta – perpendicular to the transducer – the angle is 90° and a Doppler shift can not be detected: this area is black although the flow velocity is about the same as in the ascending aorta. Further downstream, some dark blue colors indicate a low flow velocity as seen by the system, but it

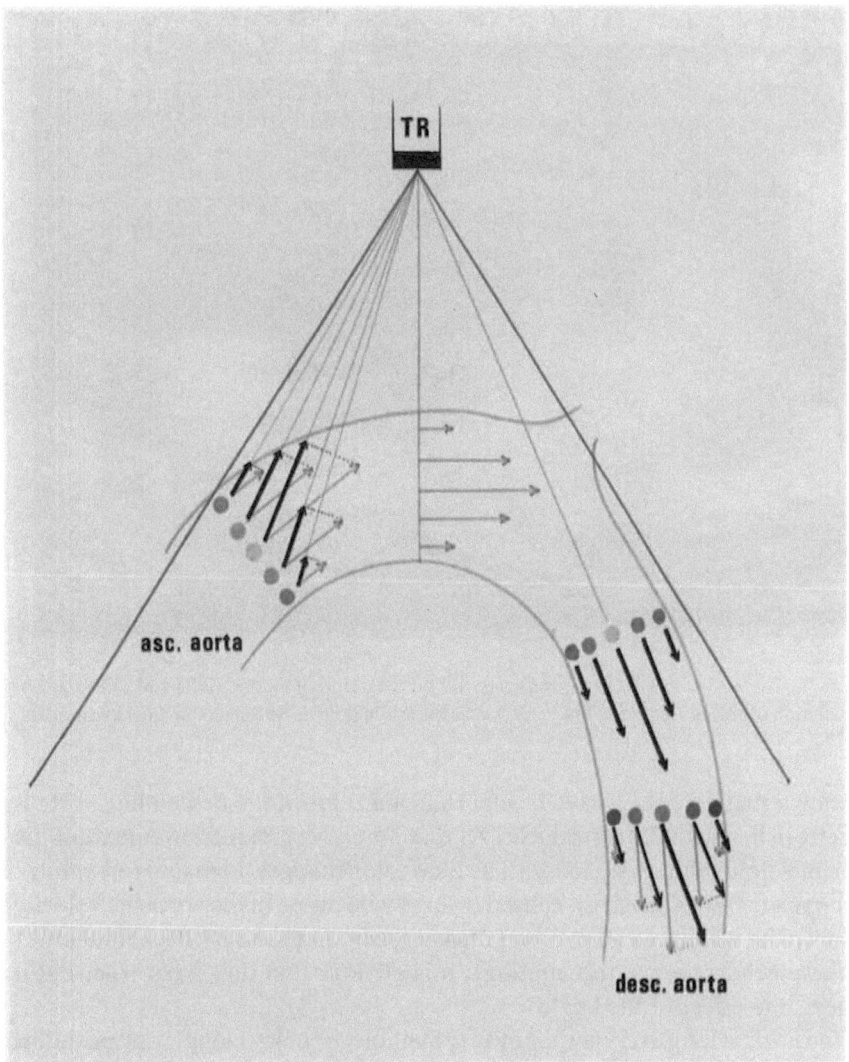

Fig. 6-10. Schematic representation of the ascending aorta, the aortic arch and the descending aorta. TR = transducer. The gray arrows indicate the well-known velocities. The black arrows show the vectors, the signals as received from the transducer. A high flow velocity towards the transducer is coded as a bright red dot, a low velocity as a dark one. A high velocity away from the transducer is coded bright blue, a low velocity dark blue. The yellow dot in the descending aorta indicates aliasing.

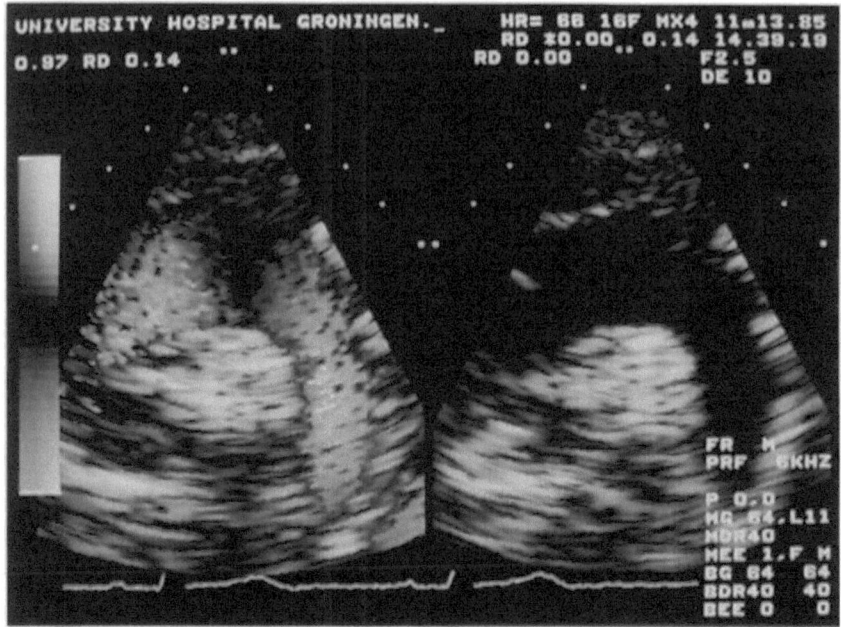

Fig. 6-11. The aortic arch from the suprasternal position during systole (left) and diastole. For explanation of colors see text of Fig. 6-10. During diastole there is no detectable flow in the aorta.

is known that velocities have hardly changed. Part of the descending aorta is exactly in line with the transducer. At that point, correct measurements of the maximal flow velocity are made. The blue color changes there into red-yellow: an opposite color (aliasing), caused by high velocities. In the aorta the velocity seems to be maximal in that area (aliasing), zero in the arch (black) and lower in the ascending aorta (no aliasing); it is obvious that this is not true, but it reflects the effect of the angle.

The normal long axis view is not very suitable for color Doppler as most flow directions are (almost) perpendicular to the Doppler sound beams (Fig. 6-12). During systole hardly any flow is recorded in the RV and the LA. The flow direction in the LV outflow tract is slightly directed towards the transducer and shows a mid-ventricular red color. The velocity augments in the area of the aortic valve (AO) where aliasing is seen. During diastole the flow direction from LA to LV is slightly directed towards the transducer and the color is predominantly red. The red flame in the RV shows inflow from the tricuspid valve. Notice several black areas in both frames: there is flow in those areas, but it is not detected with Doppler.

The normal apical view is more suitable for the detection of flow as it is predominantly directed towards and away from the transducer (Fig. 6-13).

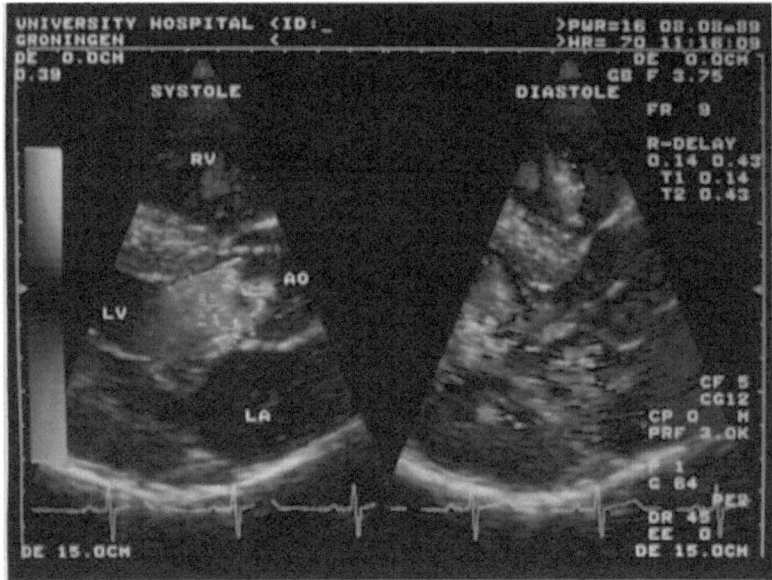

Fig. 6-12. Color flow imaging in the long axis view of a normal heart. During systole aliasing is visible at the level of the aortic valve. During diastole red colors show inflow into both ventricles.

During systole a blue color in the LV indicates a flow away from the transducer towards the aorta. At the same time the LA is filled from the pulmonary veins (red color). During diastole a red color with aliasing indicates flow through the mitral ostium. Even some turbulence is seen in the LA, caused by flow from the pulmonary veins. The blood in the LV changes in direction in the apex and turns around towards the outflow tract (blue). Colors on the right side are hardly visible as flow velocities are lower there.

Advantages of color Doppler are:
- detection of flow and flow patterns
- visualization of flow directions which includes correction of the flow velocity for the angle
- detection and localization of shunts
- distinguishing multiple lesions
- outline of endocardium
- etc.

Combined echo-Doppler examinations

Most often the Doppler examination is combined with echocardiography. This has the advantage that the position of the Doppler sound beam in the heart is

58

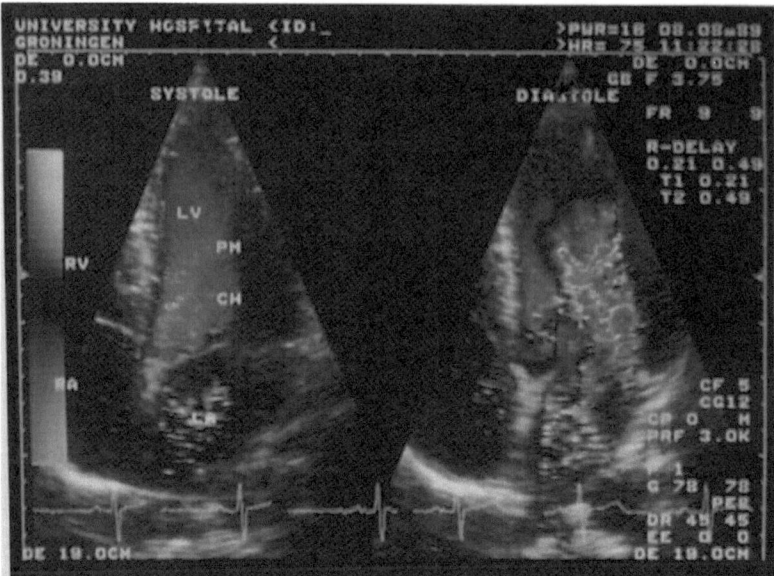

Fig. 6-13. Color flow imaging in the apical view of a normal heart. During systole a blue color indicates flow towards the aortic area. Simultaneously, red colors in the LA show inflow there from the pulmonary veins. During diastole red colors with aliasing show inflow into the LV.

visible and can be located in the area of interest.

To obtain good quality echocardiographic recordings the ultrasound beam should be directed perpendicularly to structures; for the best Doppler signals these structures often have to be parallel to the ultrasound beam. A choice has to be made in order to obtain maximal information.

Often, but especially when beginning with color Doppler echocardiography, the quickly changing colors that are visible in the moving heart are confusing. The M-mode recording is very useful then, for the timing of events. For technical reasons the colors on the M-mode recording also have a better quality than on the sector-echocardiogram.

References

Hatle L, Angelson B: Doppler ultrasound in cardiology: physical principles and clinical applications, 2nd ed. Philadelphia, Lea & Febiger, 1984.

Chapman JV, Sgalambro A: Basic concepts in Doppler echocardiography. Dordrecht, Martinus Nijhoff Publishers, 1988.

Kisslo J, Adams DB, Belkin RN: Doppler color flow imaging. New York, Churchill Livingstone, 1988.

Nanda NC: Doppler echocardiography. New York, Igaku Shoin, 1985.

Bom K, de Boo J, Rijsterborgh H: On the aliasing problem in pulsed Doppler cardiac studies. J Clin Ultrasound 12:559, 1984.

Chapter 7. Doppler examination

Introduction

The windows for combined echocardiographic and Doppler examinations are the same as for echocardiography: the left parasternal, the apical, subcostal and suprasternal positions. The positions of the patient during examinations through these windows are the same as for echocardiography.

If Doppler is used without echocardiography, the right parasternal and right supraclavicular positions are useful too. From these views, with the patient in a right lateral position, the flow in the ascending aorta can be recorded.

As with echocardiography, the gain setting of the Dopppler signal should be as high as possible. With low gain settings, weak signals may easily be missed (Fig. 7-1). On the other hand, a simultaneaous audio signal is indispensable and sometimes better than the recording on paper.

In daily practice it can be noted that there are interactions between the intensity of colors and the intensity of echoes. A high echo gain setting 'lowers' the intensity of the colors and a low echo gain setting 'intensifies' the colors (Fig. 7-2).

For optimal visualization of the flow, the color gain setting should be as high as possible, the angle as small as possible and the echo gain setting as low as possible.

The severity of under-estimation of measurement of flow velocities if there is an angle between the direction of flow and Doppler sound beam is further evaluated in Chapter 8, under right ventricle and mitral valve.

The intensity, shape and depth of color flow depend on many factors, including:
– direction of the flow
– flow velocity
– moment in the cardiac cycle
– shape of a hole

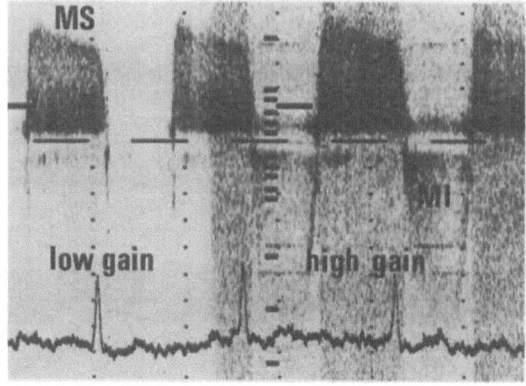

Fig. 7-1. Doppler recording from the apex in mitral stenosis and insufficiency showing the importance of gain setting. With a low gain setting only a mitral stenosis signal is recorded, with a higher gain setting also a mitral insufficiency.

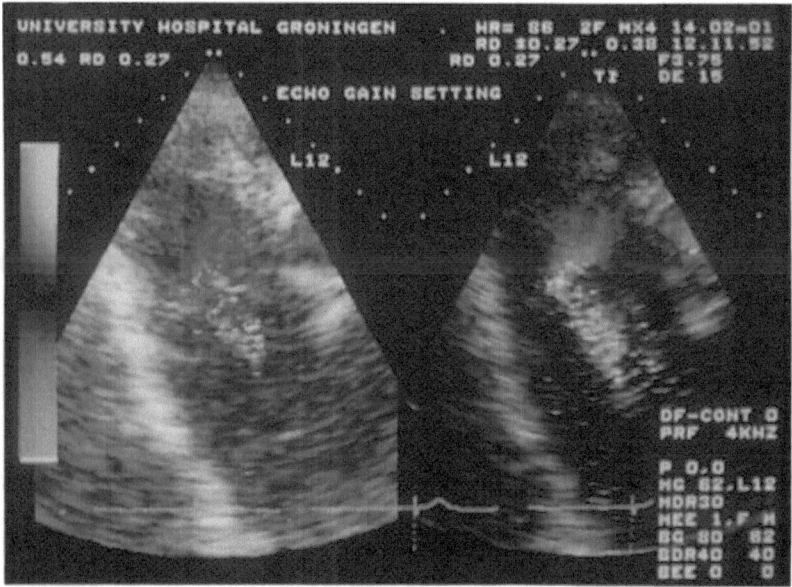

Fig. 7-2. Apical views of tricuspid insufficiency demonstrating the effect of echo-gain settings on color flow intensity. Both frames have the same color gain setting (L12). The only difference between both frames is the echo-gain setting. It demonstrates that at a high echo-gain setting, colors are less visible.

– distance from the transducer
– properties of intermediate tissue
– color gain
– echo gain
– properties of the machine
– etc.

To evaluate the severity of an insufficiency, comparisons are often made between the color flow area and the area of contrast on the angiocardiogram. The reported correlations for this comparison range from good to rather poor. In this respect it should be realized that a comparison is made between an area of visualized velocities in one plane and an area of contrast which is not necessarily representative for a volume. Not only the area of color depends on many factors, also the area of contrast on the angiocardiogram depends on several factors such as

– volume of contrast injected
– volumes of atria and ventricles
– early diastolic volume of the LV
– pressure difference
– catheter position
– viscosity of the contrast
– area of a hole
– shape of a hole
– quality of the picture (weight of the patient etc)

These variables for the color area as well as for the contrast area can make comparisons between both difficult.

Doppler recordings of the normal and abnormal aortic, mitral and tricuspid ostia as recorded from the apex and the Doppler recordings of the pulmonic ostium from the short axis aortic view are illustrated in Fig. 7 3.

The flow velocity across the normal aortic ostium starts with the opening of the aortic valve, i.e. a short time after the first heart sound (or after the R of the ECG) and later than the start of a possible mitral insufficiency. It reaches its maximum in early systole. Flow velocities from a stenotic aortic ostium are higher and show a maximum later in systole. Aortic insufficiency is recognized as starting at the end of the systolic aortic flow velocity and shows a decrease of the flow velocity during diastole. The normal mitral flow pattern resembles the M-mode recording of the mitral valve. Flow velocities are higher in mitral stenosis and the changes in flow velocities throughout diastole have usually disappeared: usually a linear decrease is recorded. Mitral insufficiency starts with the first heart sound (or the R of the ECG) and ends where the diastolic mitral inflow starts. The Doppler patterns of right sided abnormalities are the same as for left sided abnormalities.

62

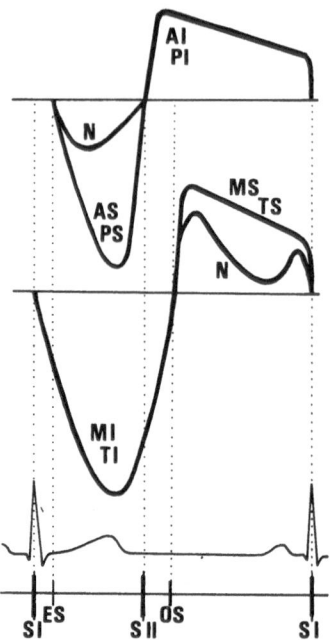

Fig. 7-3. Doppler recordings of the normal and abnormal aortic, mitral and tricuspid ostia as recorded from the apex and the Doppler recordings of the pulmonic ostium from the short axis aortic view. See text for explanation.

systolic N = normal aortic and pulmonic pattern, AS = aortic stenosis, PS = pulmonic stenosis, AI = aortic insufficiency, PI = pulmonic insufficiency, MI = mitral insufficiency, TI = tricuspid insufficiency, diastolic N = normal mitral and tricuspid pattern, MS = mitral stenosis, TS = tricuspid stenosis, SI = first heart sound, ES = ejection sound, SII = second heart sound, OS = opening snap.

Mitral valve

The apical transducer position is the best for evaluation of the flow across the mitral ostium as the flow is directed towards the transducer. The normal mitral flow resembles the M-mode recording of the normal mitral valve. A passive filling component (E) is followed by an active one, caused by atrial contraction (A). In the normal heart, the flow velocity at E is the highest (Fig. 7-4).

With color Doppler, the initial inflow into the LV is visible as a red color (towards the transducer), often with aliasing. The color intensifies again after atrial contraction. The flow is directed towards the postero-lateral wall of the LV. When turning around at the apex in the direction of the LV outflow tract it changes into blue, away from the transducer.

With TTE, mitral insufficiency can often be found with color Doppler from a normal mitral valve without the presence of a mitral insufficiency murmur. In

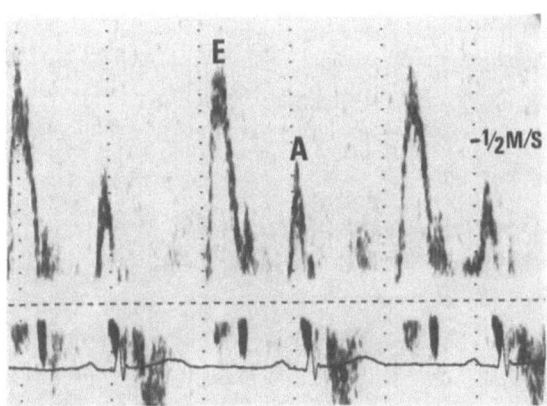

Fig. 7-4. Apical PD recording of normal mitral flow velocities. The velocities are maximal during the passive filling phase of the LV (E). The effect of atrial contraction is visible from A.

the adult, such insuffiencies are found with the trans-thoracic approach in about 40% of the normal hearts.

The esophageal approach with color Doppler however, is superior for the detection of mitral insufficiency.

Normal flow velocity at E: 0.9 (0.6-1.3) m/sec.
Normal E/A ratio ≥ 1.1.

LV outflow tract

The best transducer position for evaluation of the LV outflow tract is the apical position. With PD, flow velocities are measured 1 cm beneath the aortic valve. With CW, the velocity is difficult to measure, as from this position also the flow velocity through the aortic ostium will be measured. The flow velocity through the aortic ostium is higher than the velocity in the outflow tract and these flow velocities can not be separated with CW. This is however, not a practical problem in the use of CW: velocities in the LV outflow tract are usually only of interest if an obstruction with higher velocities than through the normal aortic ostium is expected.

With color Doppler from the apical view, the flow in the LV outflow tract of a normal heart is blue with aliasing. The aliasing is usually best seen at about 3 cm from the aortic valve. This is not necessarily the position of the highest velocity but in that region there is no angle between the direction of flow and Doppler sound beam. Thus, the machine measures the highest velocity there and not in the area just below the aortic valve: there the direction of flow has

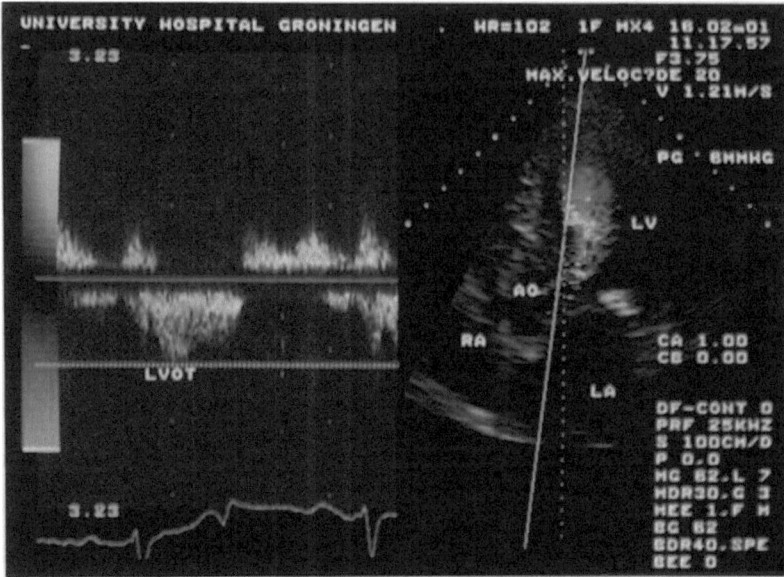

Fig. 7-5. Apical color Doppler recording of the LV outflow tract (LVOT) in a normal heart. Aliasing in the outflow tract show the highest velocities above the aortic valve: 1.2 m/sec. Velocities, however, are higher at the level of the aortic valve in the normal heart. This is not recorded because of the angle at that level and because of septal interference.

an angle with respect to the direction of the Doppler sound beam and lower velocities are recorded there than really exist (Fig. 7-5). If possible, the transducer should be placed more lateral to have the outflow tract in line with the Doppler sound beam.

TEE provides a good quality picture from the LV outflow tract. As, from the apical position, the angle between the direction of flow and Doppler sound beam, is only small, correct PD measurements can be made. The exact location of an obstruction is easily found with color.

Normal flow velocity 0.7-1.1 m/sec.

Aortic valve

The best position for evaluation of the flow velocity through the aortic ostium is the apical transducer position. For this, the transducer is placed as far as possible to the left in order to have an angle as small as possible.

From this position, the systolic flow is away from the transducer and the Doppler signal is negative (Fig. 7-6). The recording permits accurate measurements of the ejection time.

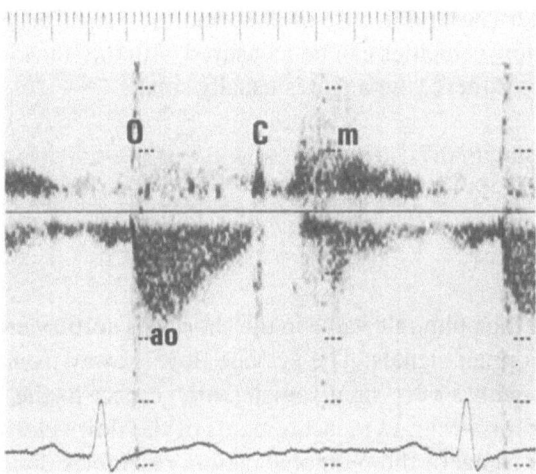

Fig. 7-6. Apical CW signal of a normal flow velocity curve (ao) through the aortic ostium. The flow is away from the transducer and starts after the end of the QRS complex. It reaches a maximum in very early systole. In this recording the reflections of the opening (O) and closure (C) of the valve also indicate that the negative signal originates from the aortic valve; it helps in differentiating from the negative signal from mitral insufficiency. Some of the mitral inflow is also visible (m) as the CW signal records al events along its beam, also the mitral inflow as recorded deeper in the LV.

The signal should be differentiated from mitral insufficiency. Mitral insufficiency starts earlier and ends later (Fig. 7-3). Also, the end of mitral insufficiency is at the same moment as the positive diastolic inflow through the mitral ostium. The audio signal is discriminative in case of weak signals.

Color flow imaging is usually not very helpful for the evaluation of the flow through a stenotic aortic valve as the aortic valve itself interferes with the ultrasound and is also rather far away from the transducer which influences the quality of the colors.

TEE may be helpful for a good visualization of the flow across the aortic ostium but is less suitable for flow velocity measurements as the direction of flow is almost perpendicular to the direction of the Doppler sound beam.

Normal flow velocity 1.3 (1.0-1.7) m/s.

Ascending and descending aorta

Flow velocities in the ascending aorta can be measured from the apical, suprasternal and right parasternal transducer positions. Often, the best signal is obtained from the suprasternal position. The best signal is also obtained by listening to the audio signals.

Color Doppler is useful in case of abnormalities, such as aortic dissection.

With TEE, flow velocities can be measured with the transducer at the level of the aortic arch: there, the angle is usually small.

Normal flow velocity 0.7-1.6 m/s.

Pulmonic valve

The position of the pulmonic valve in the short axis aortic view is ideal for the recording of Doppler signals. The systolic flow is away from the transducer without an (or with a very small) angle with respect to the Doppler sound beam. This permits accurate measurements of the flow velocity.

The Doppler signal of the pulmonic ostium resembles that from the aortic ostium (Fig. 7-3). From the Doppler signal the RV ejection time can be measured as the time from the beginning to the end of the signal. The pulmonary acceleration time is measured as the time between the beginning of the signal to the peak flow velocity. The acceleration time becomes shorter as the pulmonary artery pressure rises.

Color is helpful in localizing the maximal flow velocity through the pulmonic ostium. Very often some pulmonic regurgitation can be seen as a red color area, originating from the valve.

Because of intermediate tissue that absorbs ultrasound and the distance and large angle, TEE is not very useful for measurements of flow velocities through the pulmonic ostium.

Normal flow velocity 0.7 (0.6-0.9) m/s.
Normal peak acceleration time >110 ms.

Tricuspid valve

Tricuspid flow velocities are obtained from the short axis aortic, the apical and the subcostal views. Some 'physiological' regurgitation is often found.

Sometimes TEE can be used to measure flow velocities through the tricuspid ostium, but color is necessary then for correction of the measurement for the angle.

Normal flow velocity 0.5 (0.3-0.7) m/s.

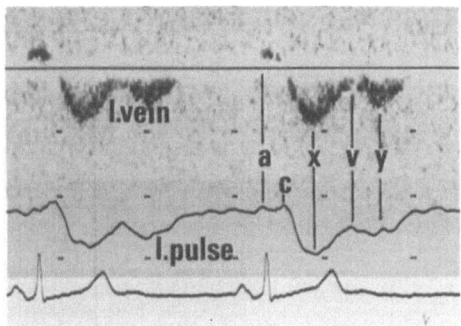

Fig. 7-7. IVC recording of the PD signal of a liver vein (l. vein) with simultaneous recording of the liver pulse ((l. pulse). a = effect of atrial contraction, c = slight ballooning of the tricuspid leaflets in early systole towards the RA, x = downward motion of the tricuspid valve during ventricular systole, v = end of filling of the RA while the tricuspid valves are closed, y = filling of the RA while the tricuspid valves are open.

SVC, IVC and hepatic veins

The supraclavicular and suprasternal positions can be used to record flow velocities from the SVC. The normal flow pattern resembles the pattern of the jugular and liver pulse recordings (Chapter 5).

From the IVC view, the IVC is perpendicular to the transducer and not suitable for Doppler measurements. The liver veins however, can be seen from this position quite well, and they are (almost) parallel to the ultrasound beam. Also from the liver veins, the Doppler signal resembles the liver pulse recording (Fig. 7-7). Especially with color, the normal regurgitation during atrial systole can be visualized very well.

References

Yoshida K, Yoshikawa J, Shakudo M, Akasaka T, Jyo Y, Takao S, Shiratori K, Koizumi K, Okumachi F, Kato H, Fukaya T: Color Doppler evaluation of valvular regurgitation in normal subjects. Circulation 78,4:840, 1988.

Sahn DJ, Maciel BC: Physiological valvular regurgitation. Doppler echocardiography and the potential for iatrogenic heart disease. Circulation 78:1075, 1988.

Hatle L, Angelson B: Doppler ultrasound in cardiology: physical principles and clinical applications, 2nd ed. Philadelphia, Lea & Febiger, 1984.

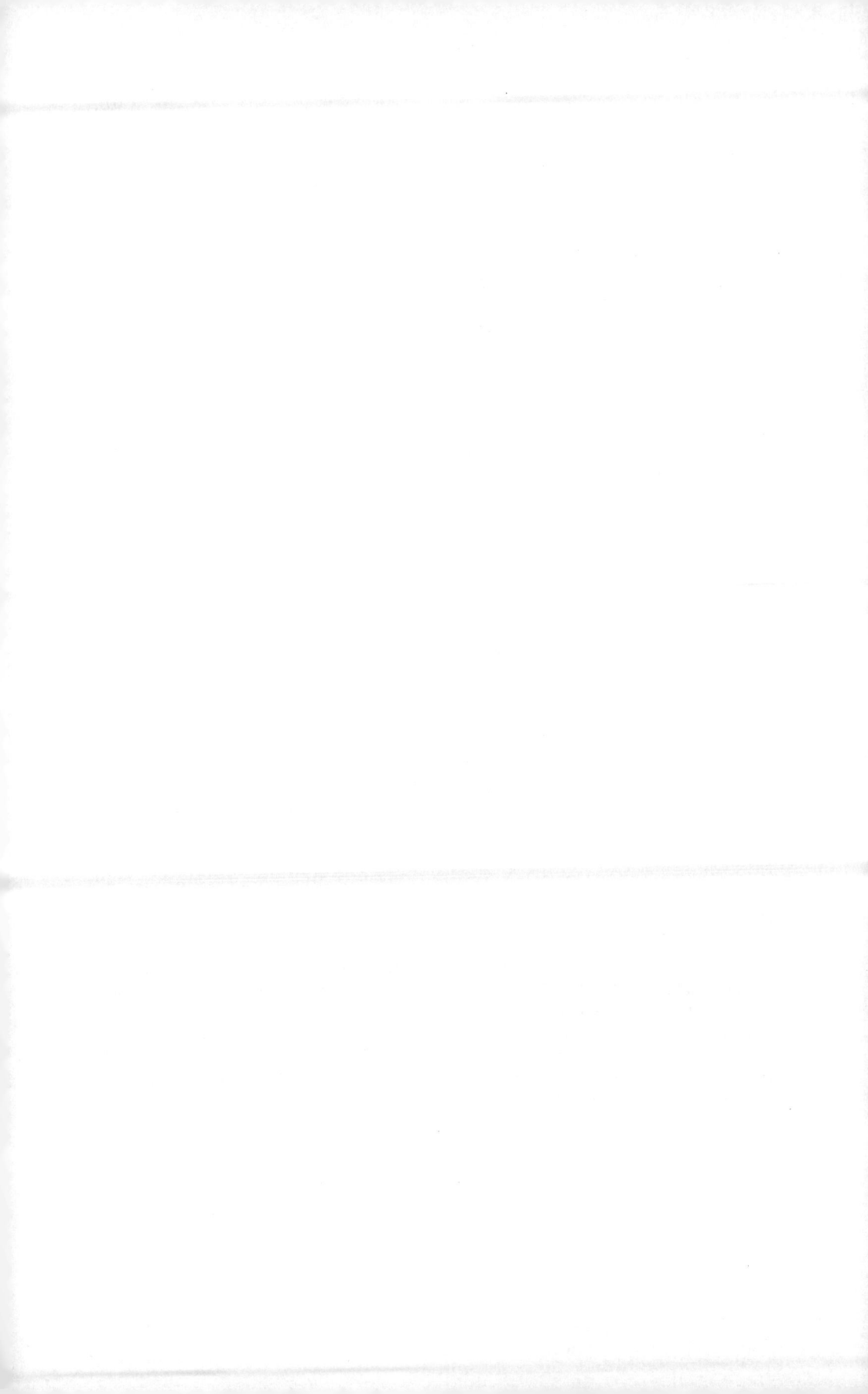

Chapter 8. Heart disease in the adult

LEFT VENTRICLE

The LV has to pump the blood through the whole body except for the lungs. Consequently, the LV has to do more work than all the other compartments of the heart together, so many indications requiring echocardiographic evaluation will concern its function. There are numerous methods for measuring the function of the LV using echocardiography, Doppler and pulse recordings.

The more often specific measurements are routinely made in the same institution, the more reliable the numbers and their interpretation will be and the more accurate the 'normal values' are for that institution. Irrespective of measurements, a description should be given of the impressions that were obtained from the sector image.

With increasing experience, there is less demand for quantitation of ejection fraction, Vcf and volumes. The combination of the other measurements mentioned below, with a description of the impressions gained is usually conclusive.

The normal left ventricle

Echocardiographic evaluation

Transducer positions
The best transducer position for visualization of the LV is the third or fourth intercostal space at the left sternal border. From this position, the ultrasound usually hits the IVS and LVPW perpendicularly (Fig. 8-1,8-2).

The apical view is used for evaluation of the apex; the endocardial outline of the other parts of the LV however, is usually poorly visible from this position: the thickness of the IVS and lateral wall, measured from the apical view, may

70

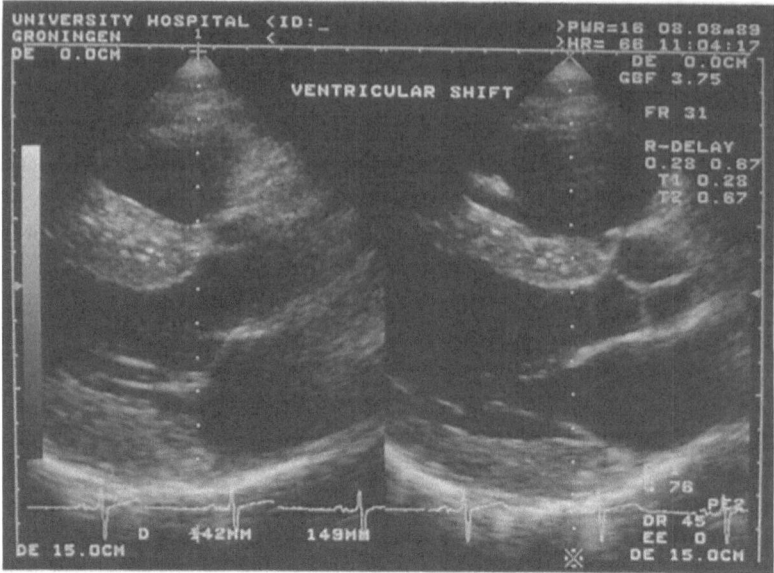

Fig. 8-1. Long axis view during systole (left) and diastole. The vertical dotted lines are in the same position in both frames. Also the transducer is in the same position and both frames are made during held expiration. Measurements of LV internal diameters, IVS and LVPW are correct from the M-mode recording of the diastolic frame. During systole however, the heart has another position (ventricular shift in apical direction) and different parts of the IVS and LVPW are then recorded.

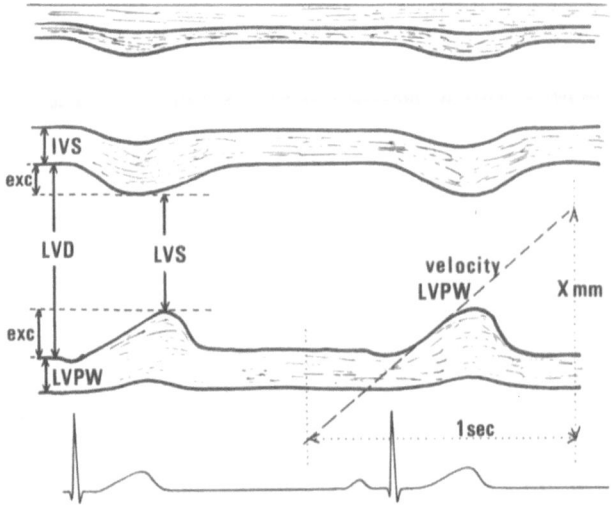

Fig. 8-2. Schematic left parasternal M-mode recording of the ventricles with the various possible measurements. LVS = systolic diameter of the LV, LVD = diastolic diameter of the LV, exc = excursion.

be severely under-estimated. This is because the ultrasound is parallel to the endocardium and reflections are poor. Usually, evaluation of the LV from the subcostal position is difficult, unless the heart is positioned low in the chest. The subcostal view is useful in patients with emphysema. Also, in these patients, parasternal evaluation is often difficult due to lung-interference.

With TEE high quality transverse sections through the LV can be obtained.

Measurements
1. LV wall thickness
2. excursion of the LVPW
3. systolic LV posterior wall velocity
4. IVS thickness
5. excursion and thickening rate of the IVS
6. LV internal diameters
7. LV 'ejection fraction' and fractional shortening
8. mean rate of circumferential fiber shortening (mean Vcf)
9. LV volumes
10. LA dimensions
11. LV ejection time, isovolumic contraction and relaxation periods
12. LA emptying index
13. M-mode pattern of the mitral valve

1. LV wall thickness
The LV wall thickness is the perpendicular distance between the endocardium and the epicardium, measured from the LVPW just below the PML. Usually, only a small part of the LVPW just below the PML and above the papillary muscles is suitable for measurement. This part can be obtained from the parasternal long axis view (Fig. 8-2,8-1). If the ultrasound beam does not transect the wall perpendicularly, wall thickness will be over-estimated (Fig. 8-3).

Most of the inner surface of the LV is rather rough caused by trabecularization. If this is included in the measurement, the thickness will also be over-estimated. Consequently, LV wall thickness should not be measured from an M-mode recording a long time after the examination, when the examiner can no longer remember if the position of the M-line was perpendicular through the ventricle. It is advisable to make measurements during the examination on the monitor or immediately after the examination from the M-mode recording. Another error in the measurement of LV wall thickness may be caused by the chordae of the PML (Fig. 8-4,8-5).

To differentiate the chordae from the endocardium, attention should be paid to the systolic thickening of the myocardium: the endocardium moves steeper during systole than the chordae. Also, if the recorded echoes remain

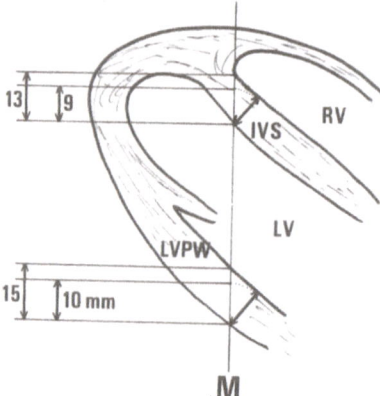

Fig. 8-3. Illustration of a cause of over-estimation of LV wall thickness if the M-line is not perpendicular to the IVS or LVPW. In this example the IVS would be 13 mm instead of 9 mm and the LVPW 15 mm instead of 10 mm.

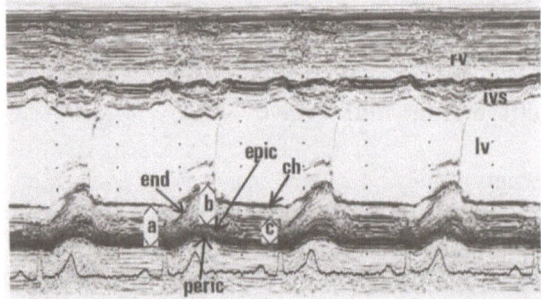

Fig. 8-4. Left parasternal M-mode recording of the RV and the LV. Distance 'a' might be interpreted as the thickness of the LVPW. The error is caused by the chordae (ch) of the PML and can be avoided by comparing 'a' with 'b', the systolic thickness of the LVPW. If both measurements are (almost) the same, there would not have been a systolic thickening, which is impossible in the presence of a good motion of the LVPW. The correct thickness is 'c'. This can usually be checked by the recording of a steeper line between the chordae and the epi/per-icardium: the endocardium (end).

parallel to the epicardium during systole and diastole, they were caused by chordae: the normal myocardium thickens during systole.

The apical area is usually difficult to record from the parasternal view. From the apical view, the apex is often too close to the usual transducer for a good recording of the endocardium. To improve the image, a higher frequency transducer can be used, such as a 5 MHz one.

If LV wall thickness is more than 11 mm, hypertrophy or amyloid may have been the cause. A thin LV wall can be caused by myocardial infarction and/or

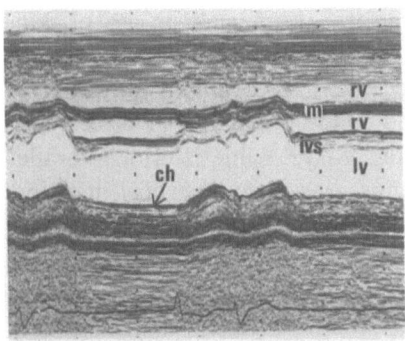

Fig. 8-5. Left parasternal M-mode recording of an ASD. During diastole the IVS shows a thickness of 10 mm. In the RV a moderator band (m) makes contact with the IVS during systole, which may cause mis-interpretation and over-estimation of the IVS thickness.

Note that the LVPW cannot be measured from this recording. The endocardium cannot be identified (see also Fig. 8-4). ch = chordae.

dilatation of the LV. Also, myocardial diseases such as dilated cardiomyopathy should be considered.

Normal LVPW thickness 7-11 mm, mean 9 mm.

2. Excursion of the LVPW

The excursion of the LVPW is the difference between the position of the endocardium during systole and diastole (Fig. 8-2). It is measured from an M-mode recording as the distance between the horizontal lines through the endocardium during systole and diastole. The distance does not represent true myocardial thickening as the epicardium also moves inward. The measurement is only reliable if the motion of the LVPW during systole is perpendicular to the ultrasound beams. This is almost always the case from the long axis view; it can be checked from the motion on the sector image.

The excursion of the LVPW is measured from the deepest position of the endocardium of the part of the LV below the PML and above the papillary muscles (usually at the a-dip, caused by atrial contraction), to the highest position during systole. A too small excursion indicates local or diffuse impairment of the myocardial function. This may be caused by e.g. infarction, ischemia, dilated cardiomyopathy and amyloid.

Normal LVPW excursion 9-14 mm, mean 12 mm.

3. Systolic LV posterior wall velocity

The systolic LV posterior wall velocity (LV velocity) shows the local systolic 'quality' of the myocardium. It is not necessarily the quality of the whole LV:

the LVPW may contract hyperkinetically in case of akinesia or hypokinesia of other parts of the LV or in the presence of mitral insufficiency. Also, posterior myocardial infarction causes local hypo- or akinesis of the LV when other parts of the LV are in good condition. The LVPW velocity is measured from an M-mode recording (Fig. 8-2). A line is drawn parallel to the endocardium during systole. This line crosses two vertical lines indicating a period of 1 second. The vertical distance between both cross-points provides the velocity in mm/second.

The measurement is especially suitable for patient follow-up.

4. IVS thickness

The thickness of the IVS is the perpendicularly measured distance between the endocardium of the RV and LV. It is usuallly measured about 2 cm below the aortic valve in the parasternal long axis view. It is not always easy or possible to obtain this view in such a way that the IVS is perpendicular to the the ultrasound beam. In that case, the measurement should be made from the frozen end-diastolic sector image, in order not to over-estimate the thickness. If the measurements are made at mid-ventricular or apical level, the thickness can be over-estimated. This is caused by the moderator band (Fig. 8-5,8-6). The moderator band is a muscular band, present in the normal RV, but more accentuated in e.g. ASD.

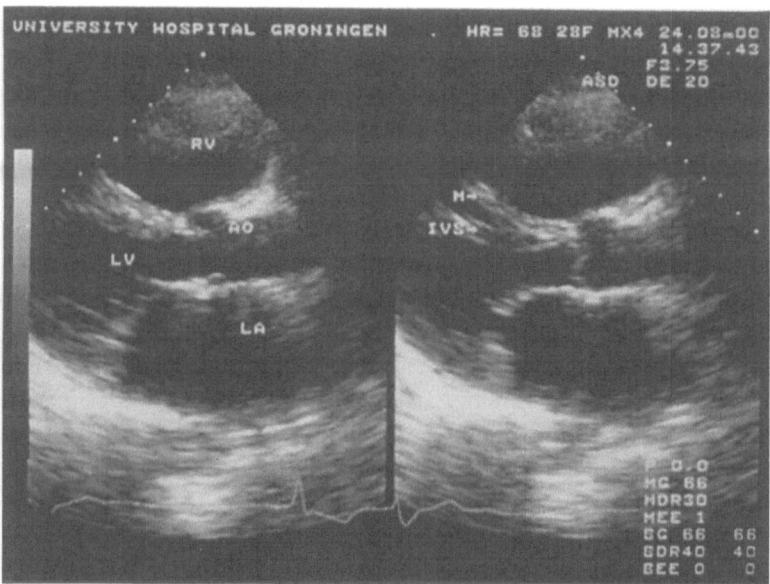

Fig. 8-6. Long axis view of an ASD. During systole (left) and diastole, the moderator band (m) may cause over-estimation of the septal thickness.

In order not to include this RV muscular band in the calculation, the short axis view of the LV is helpful for identification.

In case of a thin wall, myocardial infarction or dilated cardiomyopathy may have been the cause. In thickened IVS, diffuse (hypertrophy, amyloid) or local (sub-valvular muscular thickening) abnormalities are present.

Normal IVS thickness 7-11 mm, mean 9 mm.

5. Excursion and thickening rate of the IVS

The excursion of the IVS depends on more factors than the LVPW. Some factors are conduction disturbances and pressure and volume overload of the RV. Also, in contrast to the LVPW, the motion of the IVS is hardly ever perpendicular to the ultrasound beams from the parasternal view: the whole LV 'shifts' in apical direction during systole; with a fixed M-line, different parts of the LV are recorded during the cardiac cycle (Fig. 8-1).

The excursion of the IVS only expresses its 'contractile quality' on the M-mode if the ultrasound beam transects the IVS perpendicularly, if the function and the pressures of the RV are normal with a normal intraventricular electrical conduction and in the absence of a septal shift. This is hardly ever the case. With this in mind it is obvious that the use of the septal excursion on M-mode for the calculation of the LV internal diameters can be misleading.

To assess the 'quality' of the IVS it is useful to observe the systolic thickening. If there is no thickening at all, a myocardial infarction or HCM may be present. A poor thickening rate is seen in ischemia, HCM and amyloid.

Normal IVS excursion 3-8 mm, mean 5 mm.

6. LV internal diameters

To evaluate the size and the contraction pattern of the LV, the LV internal diameters during diastole and systole can be measured. Problems in assessing the positions of the endocardium from the LVPW and the left side of the IVS are discussed in 1,2,4 and 5.

The diameters are measured with the M-line perpendicular through the long axis of the LV, just below the aortic ring and just below the PML (Fig. 8-1). The diastolic diameter is the largest distance during diastole between the endocardium of LVPW and IVS which is most often just after atrial contraction. The systolic diameter is the shortest distance during systole between both. As maximal excursions of IVS and LVPW are not necessarily simultaneous and motion abnormalities of the IVS may be present, the systolic diameter is measured during expiration between horizontal lines through the point of maximal excursion from the IVS and LVPW (Fig. 8-2). If it is not possible to transect the LV perpendicularly, or if the middle or lower part of the IVS bulges out, sector images can be frozen during systole and diastole in order to assess the correct diameters. For follow up of patients it is advisable to document sector images with the position of the measurements in the patients file.

Normal values for the LV internal diameters for the adult differ between institutions. Even in normals, they depend on several factors such as age, body weight, heart rate, respiration, race and sex. The normal values mentioned below may be useful. One diameter however, can not be conclusive without the other: the change in diameter is important.

Normal diastolic diameter 35-50 mm
Normal systolic diameter 25-40 mm

7. LV 'ejection fraction' and fractional shortening
A good parameter to express the LV function is the ejection fraction: the percentage of blood from the diastolic volume that is ejected during systole:

$$\frac{\text{diastolic LV volume} - \text{systolic LV volume}}{\text{diastolic LV volume}} \times 100\%$$

It is misleading to think that these volumes are always represented by the LV internal diameters from the parasternal long axis view: only one dimension in one plane from only a small part of the LV can hardly be representative for the function of the whole LV. If areas from several sections are calculated (which is not always possible and also very time-consuming) the ejection fraction could be calculated.

Normal ejection fraction > 60%

Often the LV diameters from the parasternal long axis view alone are used for calculating the 'ejection fraction'. The formula above is then changed into

$$\frac{\text{diastolic LV diameter} - \text{systolic LV diameter}}{\text{diastolic LV diameter}} \times 100\%$$

This, however, is not the ejection fraction, but the fractional shortening of the LV in that particular area. With fractional shortening, no assumptions are made concerning volumes or circumferences. So long as one always remembers that only a small part of the LV is evaluated with these measurements, the formula could be used.

Normal fractional shortening 18-42%

8. Mean rate of circumferential fiber shortening (mean Vcf)
If the assumption is made that the transverse section of the LV is a circle, and that the diameters, measured from the parasternal region, are representative for this circle (which is not always correct), the mean Vcf can be calculated as

$$\frac{\text{diastolic LV diameter} - \text{systolic LV diameter}}{\text{diastolic LV diameter} \times \text{LV ejection time}}$$

The ejection time can be measured from a simultaneaous carotid pulse recording.

Normal Vcf 1.02-1.94 circumferences/second, mean 1.3 circ./sec.

9. LV volumes
To calculate the accurate ejection fraction, end-diastolic and end-systolic volumes have to be measured. For this, M-mode recordings are usually unreliable. Echocardiographic machines have the possibility of tracing the endocardium from a frozen sector image, from which an area can be calculated. Areas could also be calculated with a computer from paper recordings. The endocardium can be visualized from the parasternal long axis view, except for the apical region. However, from the apical view, the endocardium of the septal and lateral areas usually cannot be visualized as these areas are almost parallel to the ultrasound beams.

Rather reliable volume measurements are possible if assumptions are made. Described as a prolate ellipse, the LV volumes can be calculated by knowing one long axis and two minor axes. A major difficulty is that the normal LV does not have the shape of a prolate ellipse, especially not during systole. This is even worse for the abnormal LV with e.g. significant dyskinesis. A better method has been proposed by Simpson. the long axis of the LV is divided into slices of known thickness (Fig. 8-7). The sum of the slices is then equal to the volume.

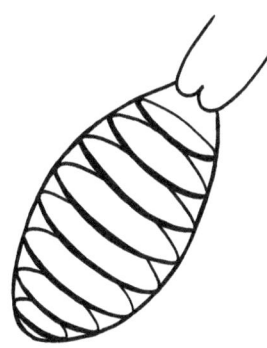

Fig. 8-7. Schematic illustration of Simpson's rule. The LV volume is expressed as a series of slices.

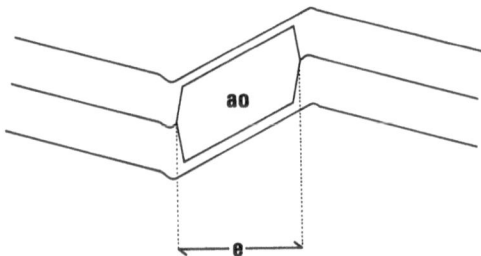

Fig. 8-8. Schematic high-speed M-mode recording of the aortic valve (ao). The ejection time (e) of the LV can be calculated as the distance between opening and closing points of the valve.

Unfortunately, this method is limited in the adult by the poor visualization of the apical region and by interference of the chest wall. Also, the method is rather time-consuming.

It should be realized that LV volumes, calculated with echocardiography, are not the same as those, measured with the isotope-technique or with angiography. Different outlines and criteria are used for these techniques.

Normal diastolic volume 95.5 ± 19.4 ml/M^2
Normal systolic volume 38.6 ± 9.5 ml/M^2

10. LA dimensions
In the absence of mitral stenosis and insuffiency, the dimensions of the LA may provide indirect information about the end-diastolic pressure of the LV. This is discussed in Chapter 8, in the section on the left atrium.

11. LV ejection time, isovolumic contraction and relaxation periods
The LV ejection time can be calculated from a recording of the aortic valve at a paper speed of 100 mm/sec. It is the horizonal distance between the points of opening and closure of the valve (Fig. 8-8). For the calculation of the ETI, the time has to be corrected for sex and heart rate (see Chapter 5). This time is exactly the same as that, calculated from the carotid pulse recording.

The isovolumic contraction and relaxation periods can be measured accurately from a dual M-mode recording of mitral and aortic valves at a paper speed of 100 mm/sec. The isovolumic contraction period is the horizontal distance between the points of mitral closure and aortic opening. The isovolumic relaxation period is the horizontal distance between the points of aortic closure and mitral opening.

12. LA emptying index
A restriction of the filling of the LV can be calculated from the LA emptying

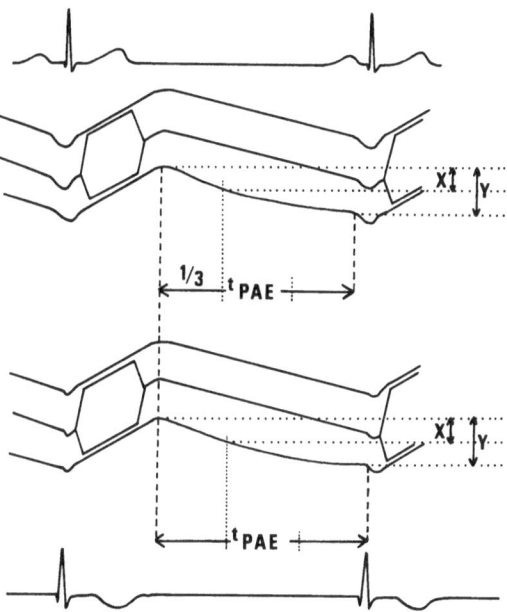

Fig. 8-9. Diagrams, demonstrating the method of calculation of the LA emptying index from the posterior aortic wall. The diastolic passive atrial emptying period (t PAE) is divided into thirds. The position of the end of the t PAE for sinus rhythm is shown in the upper diagram, for atrial fibrillation in the lower diagram. The distance x represents the downward motion of the aortic wall during the first 1/3 period, the distance y the total diastolic downward motion. If x is less than 40% of y, LV filling is restricted.

index. It is not always specific to diastolic abnormalities of the LV as impaired filling of the LV also exists in e g mitral stenosis. The LA emptying index is evaluated from the aspect of the downward motion of the posterior wall of the aorta. Normally, the LA empties rapidly with an early diastolic downward motion of the posterior wall of the aorta. If LA emptying is impaired, the aortic wall motion is reduced during the first third of diastole.

The index is calculated by dividing the diastolic period prior to atrial systole into thirds (Fig. 8-9).

In atrial fibrillation, the measurement is taken until the onset of ventricular systole. If the first third of diastole is not at least 40% of the total diastolic amplitude of the aortc wall, restricted LV filling is present.

13. M-mode pattern of the mitral valve
The M-mode pattern of the mitral valve can provide information about the LV function. This is discussed in Chapter 8, under mitral valve.

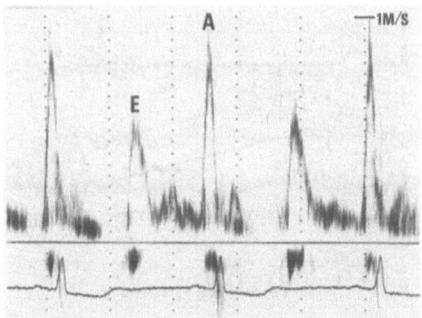

Fig. 8-10. Apical PD signal of mitral flow. The A deflection is relatively too large. The E/A ratio of 0.6 indicates an impaired LV diastolic function.

Doppler evaluation

14. flow volocities
15. estimation of the cardiac output

14. Flow velocities
The flow velocities and flow patterns through valve ostia can provide information about the systolic and diastolic function of the ventricles. Reduced early diastolic mitral flow velocities can be found in case of impaired LV compliance. Also, in ventricles with an impaired diastolic function, relatively high peak flow velocities can be found during atrial contraction (Fig. 8-10): the E/A ratio (normal value 1.1) is reduced then to values of about 0.7.

Normal values of blood flow velocities are presented in Chapter 6.

15. estimation of the cardiac output
Cardiac output is calculated by multiplying stroke volume by heart rate. The stroke volume is the volume of blood ejected by the ventricle during one contraction.

The stroke volume can be calculated from the flow velocity curves from the aorta multiplied with the cross sectional area of the aorta. The cross sectional area is calculated from the diameter of the aorta on the M-mode recording.

If the assumption is made of a flat velocity profile, the spatial mean velocity can be used. The peak velocity is integrated over the duration of systole. The resulting value is multiplied by the cross-sectional area of the aorta. At least three measurements should be made; in case of an irregular heart rhythm more than three.

For determining the stroke volume, the smallest diameter of the aortic valve ring or the diameter of the aortic arch can be used. These measurements are the main sources of error in the estimation of the stroke volume. Other errors are the assumptions that the cross-section is always circular and that the velocity profile is flat. This may be one of the reasons that good as well as poor correlations with the invasive Fick method are reported.

Pulse recordings

The value and the methods of measurements from the carotid pulse recording and the apexcardiogram for the evaluation of the LV systolic and diastolic function are discussed in Chapter 5.

The abnormal left ventricle

Local abnormalities

Wall motion
Abnormalities of the wall motion with an abnormal LV wall can be found in HCM, ischemia, myocardial infarction, aneurysm and tumors. These conditions often present in combination with an abnormal wall thickness. Therefore, HCM and tumors are discussed in those sections. Myocardial infarction and aneurysm are discussed separately.

Ischemic heart disease. In ischemic heart disease, wall thickness and thickening rate may be normal. Depending on the degree of ischemia, wall thickening can be impaired and a poor motion pattern is seen. If a normal LV wall is seen at rest, physical exertion can be used to provoke ischemia. Local abnormal thickening and hypokinesia can then be detected.
    Wall motion abnormalities of an abnormal IVS can be found in the same conditions; motion abnormalities of a normal IVS can be found in conduction disturbances and RV overload.

Conduction disturbances. Conduction disturbances such as WPW can cause abnormal motion patterns of the IVS with normal myocardial thickness and thickening rate.

RV overload. RV overload as caused by an ASD or pulmonary hypertension, may cause a paradoxical septal motion: during systole the septum moves in the direction of the RV instead of the LV.

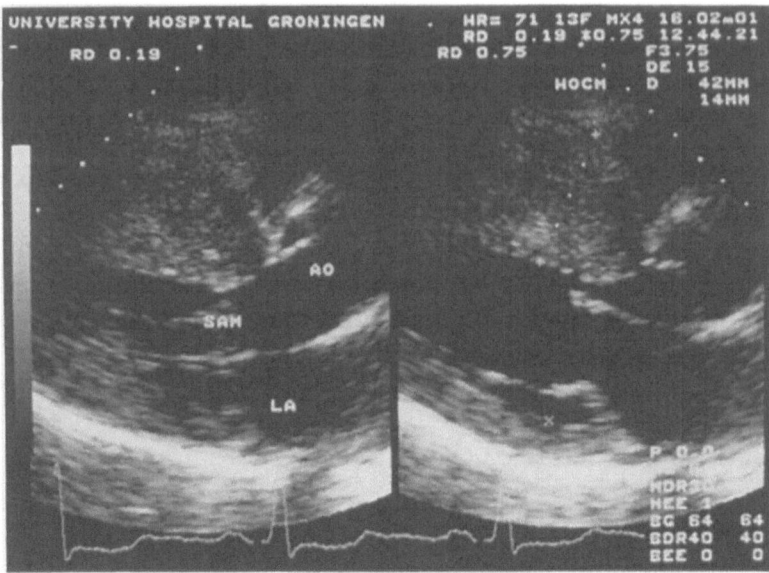

Fig. 8-11. Long axis view of HOCM during systole (left) and diastole. The IVS is greatly thickened (42 mm) and immobile. The LVPW is slightly thickened with a good contraction pattern. A systolic anterior motion (sam) shows obstruction of the LV outflow tract.

Wall thickness

Abnormalities of LV wall thickness can be found in HCM, mural thrombus, tumors and myocardial infarction.

Hypertrophic (obstructive) cardiomyopathy. Hypertrophic (obstructive) cardiomyopathy (H(O)CM) or asymmetric septal hypertrophy (ASH) or idiopathic hypertrophic sub-aortic stenosis is a primary myocardial disease. The cause is unknown. A local thickening of the ventricular wall, caused by a mass of disarranged myocardial cells is characteristic for the disease.

The complaints of a patient with H(O)CM depend on location and size of the thickening. A patient may be symptomless, but fatigue is possible as are rhythm disturbances or dizziness during physical exertion, caused by tachycardia or obstruction of the LV outflow tract. The disease is hereditary.

Because of the disarrangement of cells, there is no or hardly any systolic thickening of the involved part. It is usually located in the IVS and can then be detected from the parasternal view (Fig. 8-11). It should be noted that such a local wall thickening can be missed from the apical view (Fig. 8-12).

A local thickening of the ventricular wall can also be found in other regions than in the IVS. A location in the apico-lateral region is shown in Fig. 8-13.

The local wall thickening with loss of thickening rate can be diagnosed with

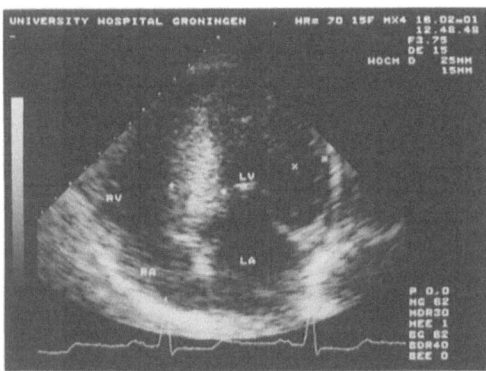

Fig. 8-12. Apical view of the same patient as in Fig. 8-11. The IVS seems to be 25 mm but is 42 mm from the long axis view. The figure illustrates that measurements of structures parallel to the ultrasound beams may be unreliable.

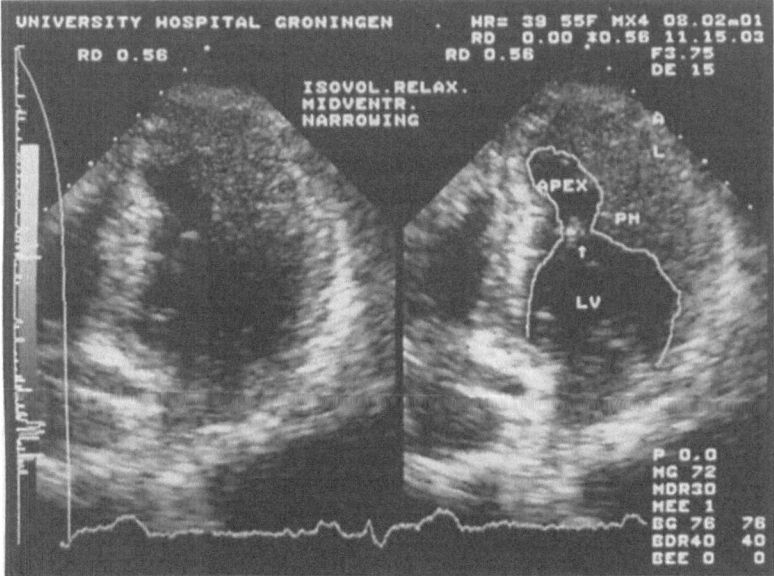

Fig. 8-13. Apical diastolic frame of HOCM, located in the apico-lateral region. The diagnosis would be missed if only a parasternal view was made. The picture is frozen during the isovolumic relaxation phase (independent of the recorded ECG!) and shows a mid-ventricular narrowing.

M-mode echocardiography. The echo-density of the local thickening is usually the same as from the normal myocardium. The local thickening can be measured and the diameter does not augment during systole. Care should be taken if a change in diameter is recorded on M-mode during the cardiac cycle. If the

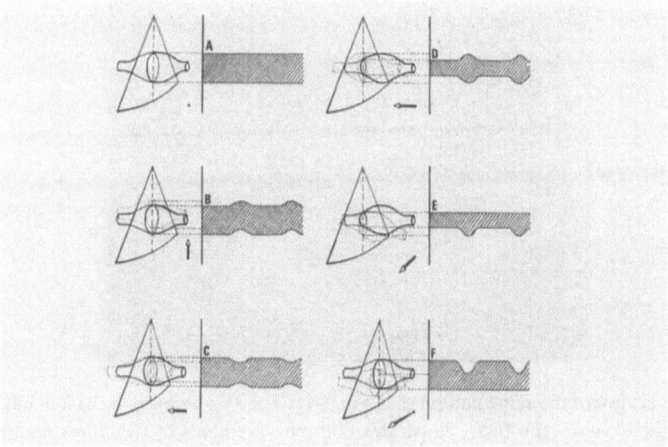

Fig. 8-14. Diagram of possible M-mode recordings from a spindle-shaped area that does not thicken or move by itself. The influence of motion of surrounding structures and the plane of section with echo are obvious and may be confusing on the isolated M-mode recording.

thickening should be spindle-shaped, Fig. 8-14 illustrates how it can be recorded on M-mode as thickening or also thinning during systole.

The result on the M-mode recording depends on the position of that area with respect to the transducer and on the motion pattern of the surrounding structures. All directions of motion can occur, not only towards and away from the transducer, but also perpendicular to it. Figure 8-14 illustrates that all possible views should be used in order to find out the spatial direction of motion of the thickened part. The short axis view of the ventricles is useful for ruling out the moderator band of the RV as a cause of 'local thickening' of the IVS. This is discussed in Chapter 8, under IVS thickness.

A classical M-mode recording of HOCM shows a thickened, hardly mobile IVS with a normal but often hyperkinetic LVPW (Fig. 8-15). However, as the IVS has no mechanical function, the remaining LV wall has to compensate for this and may be thickened by real hypertrophy (Fig. 8-16): the only difference then between IVS and LVPW is the motion pattern.

If HCM is located in the cranial part of the IVS, the outflow tract of the LV can be obstructed during systole (Fig.8-15 and 8-21). The obstruction is usually caused by the AML. Because of the narrowed outflow tract, the leaflet is drawn together with the high blood velocity in the direction of the aorta. This is called the Systolic Anterior Motion (SAM). The traction on the AML can cause mitral insufficiency (Fig. 8-21). A SAM is characterized by an anterior motion of the mitral closure line that starts at the moment of closure of the mitral valve, moves in the direction of the IVS and ends at the moment of opening of the mitral valve. The sub-valvular aortic obstruction can be severe.

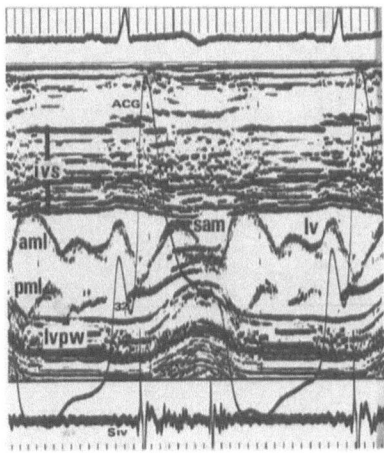

Fig. 8-15. Left parasternal M-mode recording with apexcardiogram of HOCM. The IVS is greatly thickened (34 mm) and hardly moves. The LVPW is slightly thickened (12 mm) with a good motion pattern. The LV is small. A systolic anterior motion (sam) of the AML shows obstruction of the LV outflow tract.

The a-wave of the apexcardiogram (ACG) is too large (32%), indicating increased LV end-diastolic pressure. A fourth heart sound (SIV) is recorded simultaneously with the a-wave.

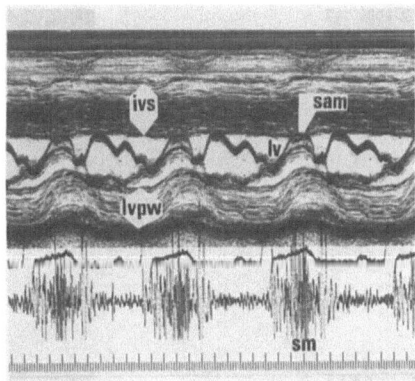

Fig. 8-16. Left parasternal M-mode recording of HOCM. The IVS is thickened (35 mm) as is the LVPW (30 mm). The difference between both is the motion pattern.

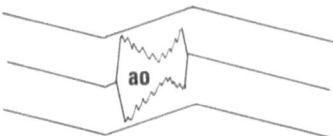

Fig. 8-17. Diagram of the motion pattern of the aortic valve in the presence of HOCM. The leaflets show a flutter and a mid-systolic tendency to close.

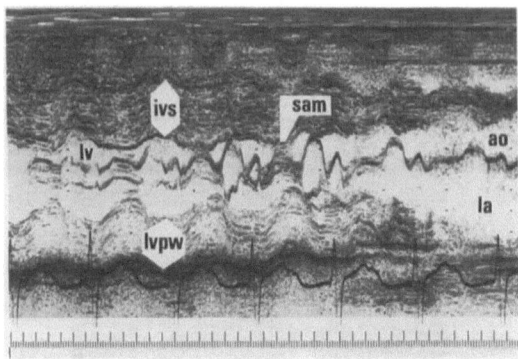

Fig. 8-18. Long axis M-mode recording of amyloid. The IVS is 27 mm, the LVPW 25 mm. The recording resembles Fig. 8-16, also a SAM is present. The difference between both recordings is the difference in motion pattern of the IVS.

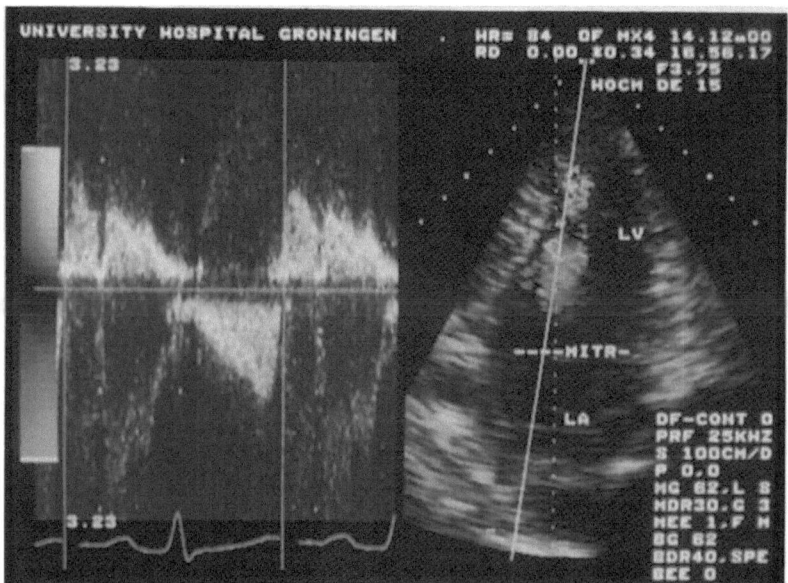

Fig. 8-19A. Diastolic apical frame of HOCM with a mid-ventricular obstruction. The red color in the LV indicates flow towards the transducer (towards the apex). Aliasing and turbulence in the apical area show an early diastolic obstruction in the LV, before mitral inflow is visible. The CW recording (left) also shows the systolic obstruction as a negative signal with a very late accent. The late accent proves augmenting severity of the dynamic obstruction caused by mid-ventricular narrowing.

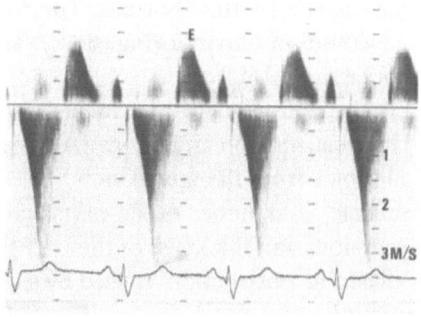

Fig. 8-19B. CW recording of a mid-ventricular obstruction in HOCM. The increase in velocity is maximal towards end-systole. The mid-ventricular pressure gradient is 43 mm Hg at a heart rate of 71 b/min. The diastolic CW Doppler recording is not representative for the mitral flow, as the Doppler beam is directed along the IVS towards the aortic ostium.

The jet in the narrowed LV outflow tract, combined with the obstruction, results in a typical systolic pattern of the normal aortic valve. The small jet causes a flutter of the aortic leaflets. Also, the usually mid-systolic obstruction causes dimished flow across the aortic ostium during mid-systole. A mid-systolic tendency to close can then be seen from the aortic valve (Fig. 8-17).

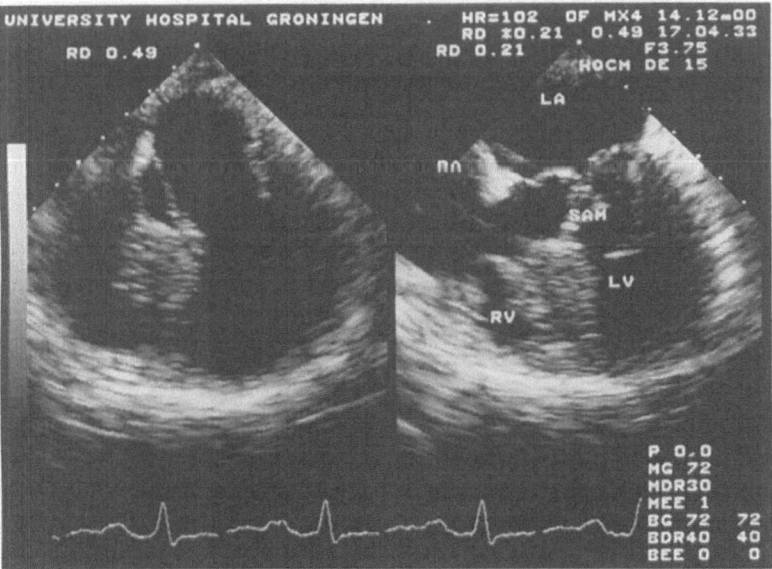

Fig. 8-20. Diastolic (left) and systolic frames with TEE of HOCM. The IVS is thickened and a SAM shows narrowing of the LV outflow tract.

88

A SAM can also be caused by the chordae. The SAM is not specific to HOCM. It can also be found in amyloid (Fig. 8-18), and in every condition with relatively long chordae.

If HCM is located in the mid-ventricular area, a muscular systolic obstruction can be found. The obstruction can be localized with color Doppler and measured with CW Doppler from the apical view.

As part of the ventricle is akinetic, other parts have to do more work. Consequently, the excursions and thickness of the LVPW are often increased.

A mid-ventricular diastolic 'obstruction' caused by a disturbed relaxation of the LV can often be found with color Doppler (Fig. 8-19).

A systolic obstruction can be measured with CW Doppler from the apical position (Fig. 8-19A,8-19B): it usually has a late-systolic accent. The obstruction is dynamic and may be absent at rest. A severe obstruction is a systolic problem to the LV and can be a reason for medical or surgical treatment. To express the severity, measurement of the obstruction alone is not enough: heart rate and the medication at the moment of measuring should also be mentioned as both greatly influence the severity of the obstruction.

The severity of the systolic obstruction however, is not the only expression of the severity of the disease. The major problem in HCM is an abnormal diastolic function, characterized by inadequate filling and impaired relaxation. The end-diastolic pressure of the LV is increased. This causes increased pressure in the LA with enlargement. The LA enlargement can also be caused by concomittant mitral regurgitation (Fig. 8-21).

The inadequate filling of the LV can be detected with Doppler measurements. From the mitral flow pattern, the early diastolic deceleration is slower. The maximal early diastolic flow velocity is reduced. The late diastolic flow

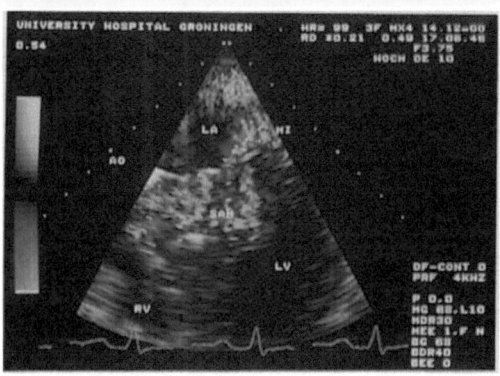

Fig. 8-21. Systolic TEE frame of HOCM. Turbulence (mixed colors) is seen at the SAM and in the LV outflow tract. The same colors are seen in the LA, showing mitral insufficiency.

velocity is increased and the ratio of early and late diastolic maximal flow velocity is often reduced (E/A ratio).

The increased end-diastolic pressure of the LV is reflected by the size of the a-wave of the ACG. The ACG recording should be a routine recording in the presence of this disease (Fig. 8-15).

With TEE excellent pictures can be obtained from the SAM and the motion pattern of the mitral valve (Fig. 8-20). Combined with color Doppler good information is obtained from the sub-valvular aortic obstruction and from the presence of concomittant mitral insufficiency (Fig. 8-21).

There is a genetic predisposition for HCM. It may be worthwhile considering whether symptom-free relatives of a patient with HCM should be investigated. There are advantages and disadvantages to such investigations. If the patient knows about the genetic predisposition, he may then be worried about children or parents. In that case the relatives should be investigated. If there are relatives with 'heart disease', murmurs, dizziness or palpitations they should also be investigated.

To be investigated in H(O)CM
echocardiography:
– wall thickness (all views)
– location of the thickened part
– thickening rate of the thickened part
– thickness, thickening rate and excursion of the remaining LV wall
– presence of a SAM (long axis, apical view)
– presence of aortic valve flutter and tendency to early closure (long axis view)
– LV dimensions (long axis view)
– LA dimensions (long axis, apical view)
Doppler:
– systolic intraventricular pressure difference (apical view)
– mitral insufficiency (apical view)
– mitral flow pattern (apical view)
color Doppler:
– indirect outline of the endocardium (apical view)
– location of intraventricular obstruction (apical view)
pulse recording:
– a/H ratio from the ACG

Thrombi. Mural thrombi can be found in the LV in akinetic areas, caused by a myocardial infarction (Fig. 8-22).

A thrombus mass can have various shapes. It is recognized as a mass of echoes located at an akinetic area. Most often, the echo-density of a thrombus

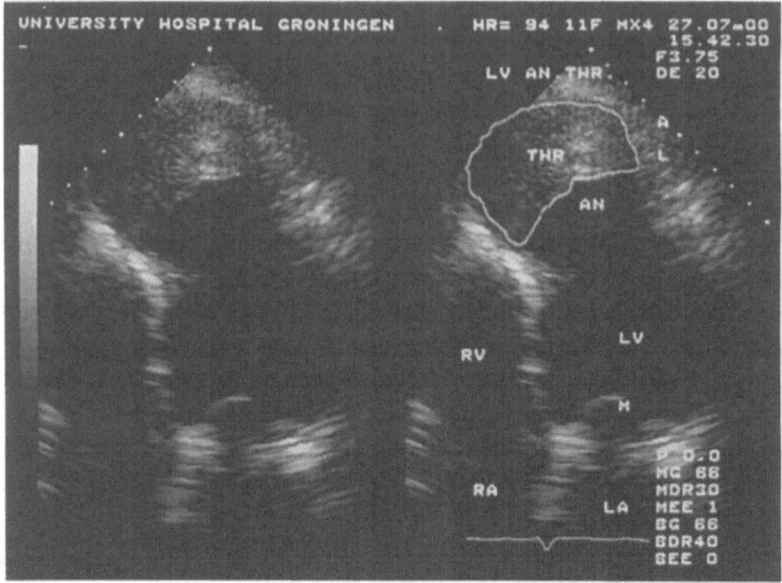

Fig. 8-22. The apical view of a LV aneurysm (AN) after inferior myocardial infarction. A thrombus (THR) fills up almost the whole aneurysm.

mass is about the same as that from normal myocardium. A flat and thin thrombus mass can hardly be distinguished from the real LV wall. A false interpretation may then be made of a thickened and akinetic part of the LV wall. LV thrombi are also discussed in Chapter 8, in the section on 'intracardiac masses'.

Tumors. Tumors of the LV are rare. Direct invasion of the LV wall by a tumor can cause increased local echo-density with decreased wall motion (Fig. 8-23). LV tumors are also discussed in Chapter 8, section 'intracardiac masses'.

Myocardial infarction and aneurysm

In classical myocardial infarction, part of the ventricle is thin-walled (2-5 mm) and akinetic. The echo-density from the infarcted area is often higher than that from the surrounding normal myocardium.

The echocardiographic image depends on location and extent of the infarction. A small, non-transmural infarction can hardly be seen. In small transmural infarctions, only 'hypokinesis' may be visible. This is not activity from that part of the myocardium itself: the contracting surrounding myocardium takes the infarcted area with it in its motion. Large infarctions, especially if hit perpendicularly by the ultrasound, are seen as local akinetic, thin walls.

If part of the LV is akinetic, other parts have to compensate for this loss of

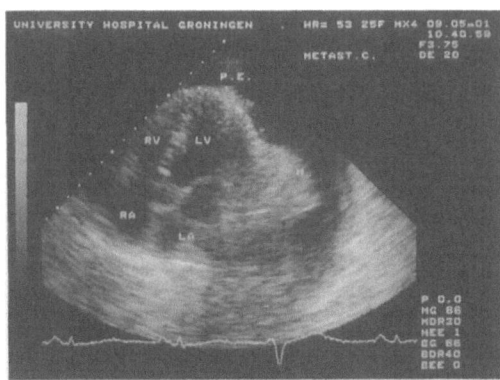

Fig. 8-23. Apical view of invasion of LV and LA with a metastatic carcinoma (M) of the lungs. As is often the case in metastatic carcinoma, pericardial effusion (P.E.) is present.

function and may show hyperkinesis. If in large myocardial infarctions, hyperkinesis of the remaining myocardium cannot be found, the non-infarcted myocardium may have a relatively poor contraction pattern caused by diffuse myocardial abnormalities or by ischemia.

In large myocardial infarctions, the LV may be dilated. Depending on localization of the infarction, measurements should not only be made from the standard positions of the parasternal long axis view. For example, in septal infarction, the diameters between IVS and LVPW are not necessarily representative for the whole LV: the apical region may show a vigorous contraction pattern. Also, more coronary vessels may be abnormal and the apical area shows a poor contraction pattern. So, a careful description of the motion pattern of the remaining heart should also be given.

Local dysfunction of the LV wall by myocardial infarction or ischemia, is often the cause of mitral insufficiency. This again causes LA enlargement. Another reason for LA enlargement is increased LVEDP that can exist in impaired LV function, caused by myocardial infarction. This may cause pulmonary hypertension, measurable with color Doppler and CW in the presence of tricuspid insufficiency.

Major complications of myocardial infarction are rupture of the IVS and rupture of a papillary muscle. The clinical differentiation between both can be difficult. Both are serious complications for which immediate surgery is often needed. They can be differentiated with echocardiography, but a quick diagnosis can be made with color Doppler (Fig. 8-24).

Rupture of the IVS shows an akinetic or hypokinetic area from the IVS. Sometimes the rupture can be seen directly on the echocardiogram. The IVS still has its normal thickness, as rupture usually occurs within less than 3 days after infarction; there has not yet been time for the myocardium to become

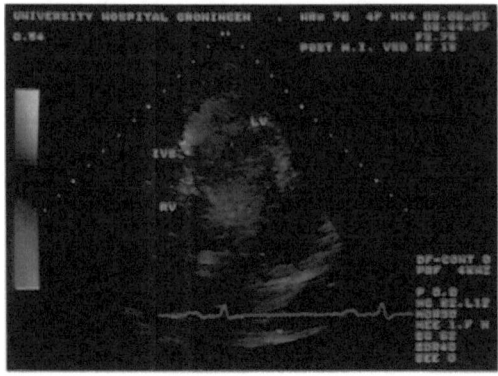

Fig. 8-24. Apical systolic frame of a VSD after myocardial infarction. The IVS bulges out to the RV. A blue color with aliasing at the IVS indicates a flow from the apex of the LV to the rupture in the IVS.

organized into connective tissue and thus become thinner. However, a systolic thickening is absent. Direct visualization of the rupture can be difficult, but the shunt is easy to detect with color Doppler. Papillary muscle rupture can be seen directly. Often indirect features are present, such as a flail part of the mitral valve. The massive mitral insufficiency can easily be found with Doppler.

Another complication of myocardial infarction is the development of an aneurysm. Three types of aneurysms can be distinguished: true, saccular and false aneurysms (Fig. 8-25).

A true aneurysm is a diffuse outward bulging of an akinetic or dyskinetic LV wall. As flow velocities in an aneurysm are low, thrombi are often found there. A flat thrombus against the wall may cause over-estimation of wall thickness when the thrombus is included in the calculation. However, this is not a real problem as the aneurysm itself has already been recognized. An aneurysm can be blown up like a balloon, sometimes with a relatively small connection with the LV: a saccular aneurysm. Incomplete rupture of the free wall of the LV is also possible following myocardial infarction. Thrombi, together with pericardium, keep the process local. These false aneurysms communicate with the LV through a small hole (Fig. 8-26A, 8-26B). The wall of a false aneurysm has no myocardial fibres. With echocardiography they sometimes can hardly be differentiated from saccular aneurysms.

The extent of an aneurysm should be described and measured. If surgical resection is considered, the position of the papillary muscles with respect to the aneurysm should also be described.

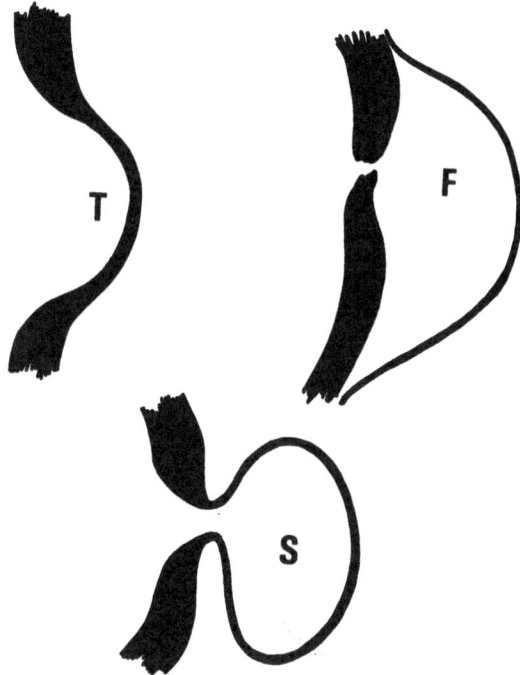

Fig. 8-25. Types of aneurysms. T = true aneurysm, the ventricular wall bulges out and is akinetic or dyskinetic. F = false aneurysm, following incomplete rupture of the ventricular wall. There are no myocardial fibers in the wall of a false aneurysm. S = saccular aneurysm, a blown up part of the ventricular wall, connected with the LV with a small hole.

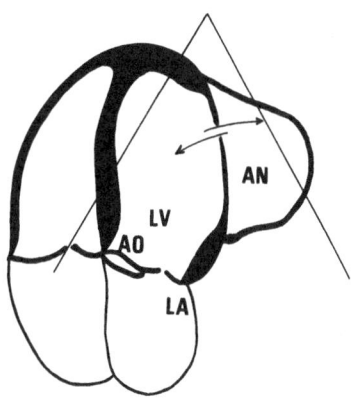

Fig. 8-26A. Apical view of the LV with a false aneurysm. The drawing illustrates how the flow enters and leaves the aneurysm during systole and diastole.

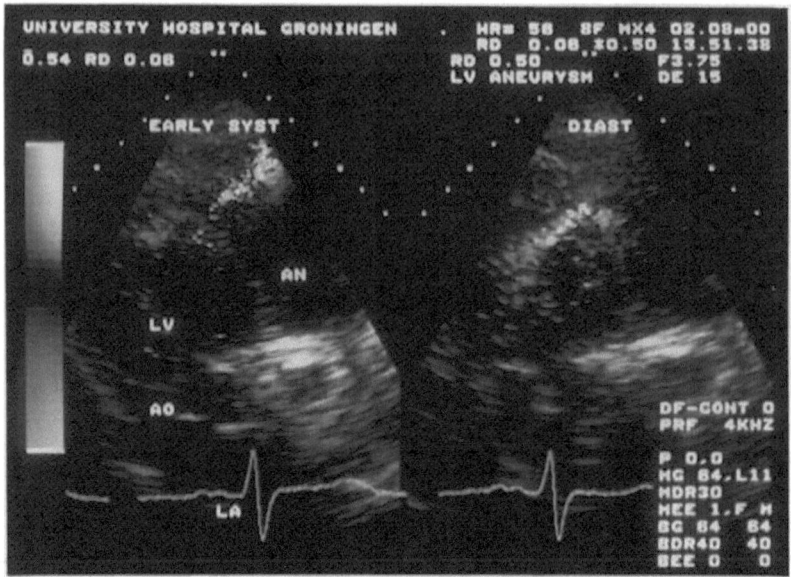

Fig. 8-26B. Apical view of the LV with a false aneurysm. The section is explained in Fig. 8-26A. On the left a red color indicates a flow into the aneurysm, on the right it leaves the aneurysm again, indicated by a blue color with aliasing.

To be investigated in myocardial infarction/aneurysm
echocardiography:
– LV wall thickness, dimensions (long axis view)
– LA dimensions (long axis, apical view)
– extent of the infarcted area
– hypo-, a-, or dyskinesia
– thrombus masses
Doppler:
– mitral insufficiency (apical view)
– tricuspid insufficiency (apical view, short axis aortic view)
color Doppler:
– RV peak pressure from tricuspid insufficiency
pulse recording:
– a/H ratio

Diffuse abnormalities

Wall thickness abnormalities can often be found in combination with wall motion abnormalities. Therefore, they will both be discussed in the following.

A normal wall thickness with a poor motion pattern is often found in situations of dilatation of the LV after a period of some hypertrophy. This LV failure can be caused by e.g. severe mitral insufficiency and aortic insufficiency and occasionally by a large VSD or PDA.

A normal wall thickness with a good motion pattern can be found in LV volume overload such as mitral and aortic insufficiency and in people practising intensive sports.

A thin wall with a poor motion pattern is usually found together with an enlarged LV (Fig. 8-27).

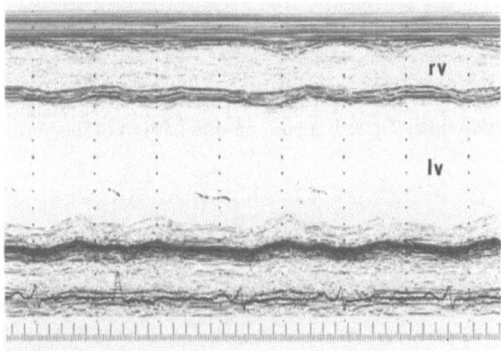

Fig. 8-27. Left parasternal M-mode recording of a dilated cardiomyopathy. IVS as well as LVPW are thin and have a poor motion pattern. The LV is enlarged.

In the absence of valvular heart disease the myocardium itself can be the cause. Such a DCM picture may have had many causes. In DCM, wall thickness is usually less than 8 mm with poor excursions (hypokinesis) and a poor thickening rate. The LA is enlarged by an increased LVEDP and by mitral insufficiency. Mitral insufficiency is usually present and is caused by dilatation of the LV or sometimes by dilatation of the mitral valve ring. The peak flow velocity in the ascending aorta succesfully discriminates between patients with DCM and normal subjects without overlap and also with the echocardiographically measured Vcf.

The ejection time is shortened. It can be calculated from the recording of the aortic valve (Fig. 8-28).

As the LV has lost much of its 'contractile force', the flow velocities will be low with a small stroke volume. This is often reflected by the aortic valve, sometimes by a poor cusp separation, often with a tendency to close that can start already in early systole. The closure velocity of the aortic valve is decreased (Fig. 8-28). Also, the aortic root has a poor motion pattern, a reflection of the low cardiac output. The diastolic flow velocities are also decreased. This is reflected by a poor separation of the mitral leaflets and low flow velocities across the mitral valve (Fig. 8-29).

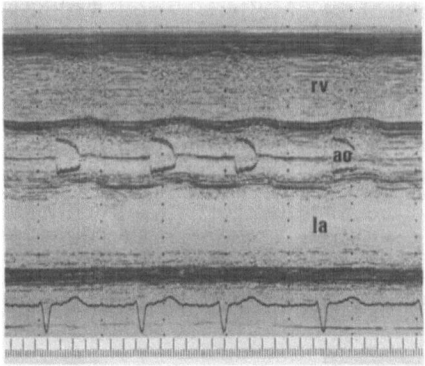

Fig. 8-28. The aortic valve (ao) in DCM. There is an early tendency to close and also early closure with a shortened ejection time. There is a poor motion pattern of the aortic root.

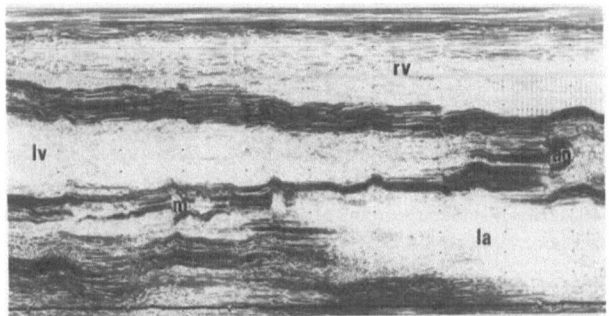

Fig. 8-29. Left parasternal M-mode sweep of a patient with a cardiomyopathy. The LV is enlarged with a poor contraction pattern. The LA is enlarged by the increased LV end-diastolic pressure and/or mitral insufficiency. Note the poor separation of both the aortic and mitral valve, caused by a small stroke volume.

Low flow velocities may cause thrombus masses in the heart. Transmitral flow velocity is lower in DCM but also in hypertension. The late flow velocity is unchanged in DCM compared with normals. The results, however, depend on the absence or presence of mitral regurgitation.

There are several causes for a DCM-like picture. It can be found in severe, almost diffuse ischemic heart disease and also post-myocarditis.

To be investigated in DCM
echocardiography:
– LV wall thickness, dimensions (long axis view)
– is wall thickness uniform? (all views)
– thrombus masses (all views)

- early closure of the aortic valve? (long axis view)
- LA dimensions (long axis, apical view)
- diameter of the IVC during respiration
- optional: all other measurements of the LV

Doppler:
- flow velocities
- mitral insufficiency
- tricuspid insufficiency

color Doppler:
- RV peak pressure from tricuspid insufficiency

pulse recording:
- a/H ratio

A thick wall with a good motion pattern of the LV is caused by overload, especially pressure overload (hypertension, sub-valvular, valvular and supra-valvular aortic stenosis, coarctation) (Fig. 8-30). If dense echoes are found from the aortic valve, together with a thick-walled LV with a good motion pattern, the aortic valve should be examined with Doppler for the presence of aortic stenosis. Several patients with unsuspected severe aortic stenosis have been discovered this way!

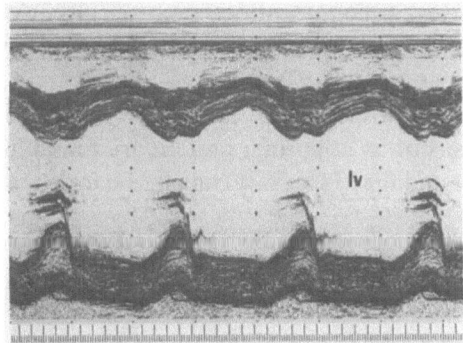

Fig. 8-30. Left parasternal M-mode recording of a typical pattern of LV hypertrophy: a thickened IVS and LVPW, both with a good motion pattern. The LV is also enlarged.

A thick wall with a poor motion pattern can be found in long standing severe hypertension with LV failure. Then, the LV dilates with decrease of the motion pattern. This condition may be difficult to distinguish from amyloid. With further dilatation even a DCM-like picture can be found, but with a normal or thickened wall. In severe aortic stenosis, failure of the LV also results in decrease of motion pattern and in dilatation. In very severe aortic stenosis the systolic-diastolic difference can be poor in the presence of a good

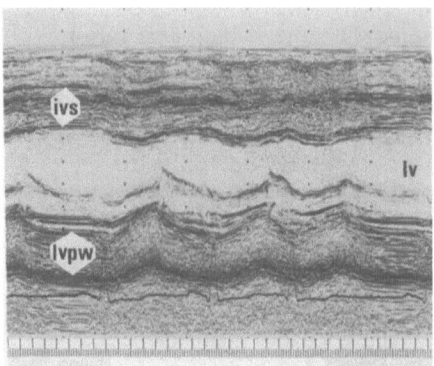

Fig. 8-31. Left parasternal M-mode recording, showing thickening of both IVS and LVPW. The contraction pattern is not optimal and the picture should not be confused with amyloid. This rather poor contraction pattern was caused by severe aortic stenosis.

quality LV (Fig. 8-31). The picture is suggestive then for a poor quality LV. The echocardiographic findings of aortic stenosis will be discussed in more detail in Chapter 8, the section on the aortic valve.

A thick-walled LV with a poor motion pattern can also be caused by amyloid and other infiltrative cardiomyopathies such as glycogen storage disease (Pompe's disease), hemachromatosis and sarcoidosis. The most common type is amyloid heart disease (Fig. 8-32).

Long standing infectious diseases can be the cause for amyloid. In this abnormality, deposits of an abnormal protein are found in parenchymatous organs like the liver and the kidneys. It can also be found in the myocardium,

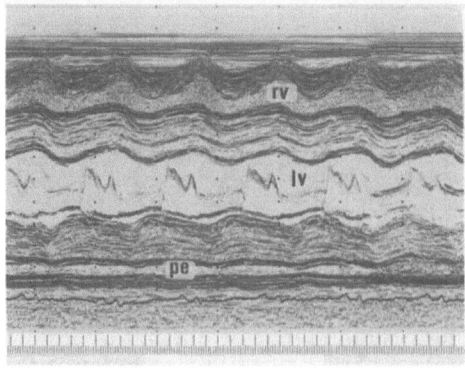

Fig. 8-32. Left parasternal M-mode recording of amyloid. The LV walls are thickened and have a poor contraction pattern. The LV diameters are rather small. The thickened RV anterior wall supports the diagnosis of amyloid. Some pericardial effusion (pe) is seen behind the LV.

but the heart is not always involved in amyloid. The protein deposits suppress the myocardial function.

As in amyloid both systolic and diastolic functions are impaired, and the patient complains of fatigue and shortness of breath during physical exertion or even at rest.

Patients with amyloid often have exceptionally clear echocardiograms. The echoes are usually brighter than normal (Fig. 8-33). This high echo density is also helpful in discriminating amyloid from LV failure by other causes.

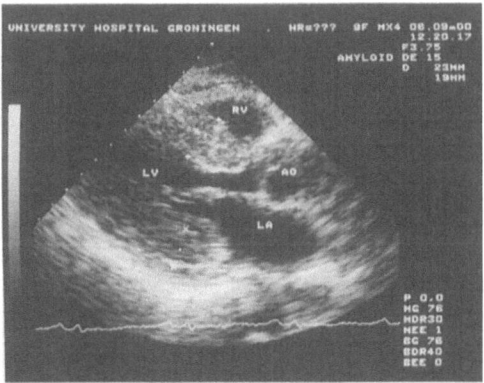

Fig. 8-33. Left parasternal view of amyloid. The walls of IVS and LVPW are equally thickened. The RV wall is also thickened. There are bright echoes from all structures.

As amyloid of the heart involves the whole heart, the RV anterior wall may also be thickened. The motion pattern in amyloid is poor, the ejection time is shortened. This is reflected by the low output aspect of the aortic valve with an early tendency to close (Fig. 8-28). Often, the valves are also echogenic and thickened (Fig. 8-34).

Two types of cardiac involvement can be found in amyloid. The classical type is the type in which the external diameters of the LV are normal and the internal diameters small. We found systolic diameters of the LV in this situation of 5 mm. The other type can show normal brightness of the echoes with dilatation of the LV.

Other diseases with myocardial involvement

In endomyocardial fibrosis, the picture of a congestive cardiomyopathy or a restrictive cardiomyopathy may be found with impaired LV filling. Dense echoes may be found from the endocardium (Fig. 8-35). However, we also found a normal echocardiogram from a patient who at autopsy a few days later had an endocardium 3 mm thick.

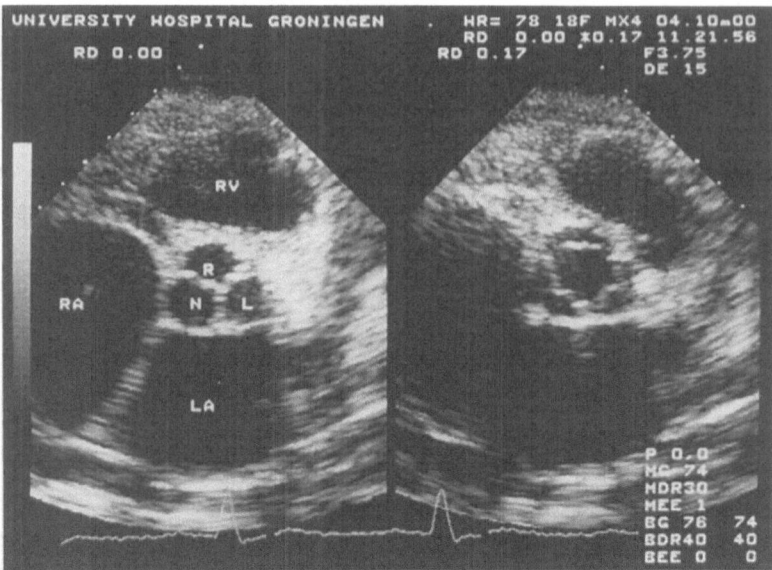

Fig. 8-34. Short axis aortic view of amyloid. The echogenicity is rather characteristic of the disease: all three cusps of the aortic valve are identified clearly in this elderly patient. R = right coronary cusp, L = left coronary cusp, N = non coronary cusp.

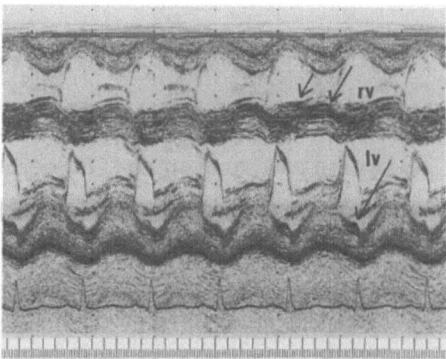

Fig. 8-35. M-mode recording of endomyocardial fibrosis. A few echogenic areas are visible from the right side of the IVS and from the LVPW.

In Friedreich's ataxia LV dysfunction can be present. A thickened LV wall may be found (Fig. 8-36), resembling amyloid. Many other neuromuscular disorders are associated with LV function disturbances. They are often seen as DCM-like pictures.

In acromegaly, cardiomegaly with LV hypertrophy may be found, but dilatation has also been described. Occasionally, the picture can resemble

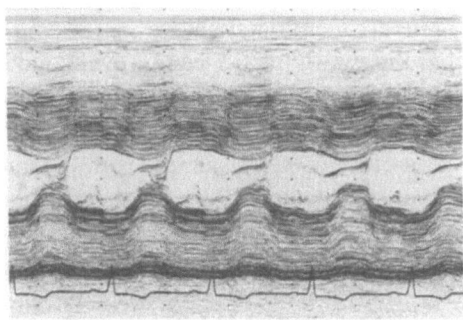

Fig. 8-36. Diffuse thickening of the LV in Friedreich's ataxia. The picture resembles that of amyloid.

HCM. The systolic LV function is usually normal.

In hypothyroidism LV dilatation and decreased systolic function can be found that may revert to normal after treatment.

RIGHT VENTRICLE

The normal right ventricle

Echocardiographic evaluation

Because of the position of the RV with respect to the chest wall, echocardiographic imaging is not as simple as from the LV. Much of the RV is just under the sternum, preventing the recording of echocardiographic images. The RV is not globally shaped as is the LV, and estimation of the volume is not reflected well by M-mode measurements. Also, the internal diameters in specific directions, change with the position of the patient. Wall thicknesses are often difficult to measure except with higher frequency transducers from the parasternal region.

From the parasternal view, the RV anterior wall is the first moving structure that is recorded. As it is close to the transducer, it can be investigated better with a 5 MHz transducer. Behind the RV anterior wall, only a small part of the volume of the RV can be seen. Measurements of the RV can be made from this position from the inner surface of the RV anterior wall to the right side of the IVS. This measurement is usable but hardly reflects the RV volume.

From the subcostal position, the RV wall thickness can often be measured better than from the parasternal position: the wall is at a greater distance and more of it can be seen in one plane. Normal RV wall thickness is not exactly known; we use the numbers mentioned below.

From the apical view the size of the RV can be evaluated better. The size of the RV can be compared with that of the LV. In the presence of a normal LV, the normal RV is smaller. Wall thickness is difficult to measure from this position as the direction of ultrasound is in line with the endocardium.

Efforts have been made to calculate RV volumes. Calculations are not very accurate, difficult and time consuming to make. In routine echocardiography, estimation of the RV volume is made from several transducer positions.

Normal RV wall thickness less than 4 mm
Normal RV dimension from the parasternal view 7-23 mm, mean 1.5 mm

Doppler evaluation

Attempts have been made to calculate the output of the RV non-invasively. This is important for the evaluation of the severity of shunts. The output can be calculated if the flow through and the diameter of the pulmonary artery are known. The principle of output measurement is described in Chapter 8, on the left ventricle.

The abnormal right ventricle

Right ventricular overload

As pressure and volume overload of the RV have various effects with various echocardiographic features, they are discussed separately. Combinations of both are often secondarily caused by e.g. LA overload such as in mitral valve abnormalities, increased LVEDP and obstructing LA tumors.

Volume overload. Volume overload of the RV is caused by ASD, abnormal venous drainage, tricuspid insufficiency, and pulmonic insufficiency. Important volume overload results in RV dilatation. Another feature of volume overload is the abnormal motion pattern of the IVS: during ventricular systole the IVS moves towards the RV instead of towards the LV (Fig. 8-5). This paradoxical IVS motion pattern is usually found in RV volume overload but may also be found in pure and severe RV pressure overload.

Pressure overload. Pressure overload of the RV is caused by sub-valvular and valvular pulmonic stenosis and by pulmonary hypertension. It causes RV wall thickening with a good motion pattern. In severe pressure overload, the geometry of the LV can be distorted by displacement of the IVS (Fig. 8-37).

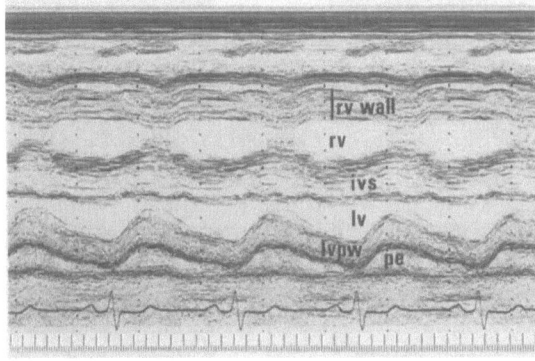

Fig. 8-37. Left parasternal M-mode recording of a long standing severe pulmonary hypertension. The RV wall is greatly thickened (19 mm) as is the IVS. The LVPW is slightly thickened. The LV internal diameters are exceptionally small. There is some pericardial effusion (pe) behind the LVPW.

Wall thickness

A thickened RV wall can be found in pressure overload and in various diseases such as Löffler's endocarditis (Fig. 8-35) and in amyloid (Fig. 8-32). In amyloid the echoes are brighter and there is a poor motion pattern of the wall. Also, the LV wall is thickened in amyloid. This aspect of RV wall thickness can be helpful in evaluating the cause of diffuse LV wall thickness and discriminate between general myocardial disease and LV abnornalities.

Moderator band, double-chambered RV, sub-valvular pulmonic stenosis

In RV overload, the moderator band of the RV may be thickened. From the parasternal short axis view of the ventricles this band can be identified as a band, originating from the anterior part of the IVS.

In muscular sub-valvular pulmonic stenosis, the outflow tract of the RV is narrowed. This is diagnosed from the short axis aortic view. Effects of the narrowing are found on the pulmonic valve: a flutter and sometimes an early tendency to close are recorded.

Occasionally, a sub-valvular stenosis can be present low in the RV. The RV is separated then in a caudal and cranial part. A pressure gradient can be found between 'both' RV chambers (double-chambered RV). The stenotic area divides the RV into two parts.

In sub-valvular stenosis and in double-chambered RV the combination of both color Doppler and CW Doppler is valuable for establishing the diagnosis and the severity of obstruction. Color Doppler is especially helpful for the

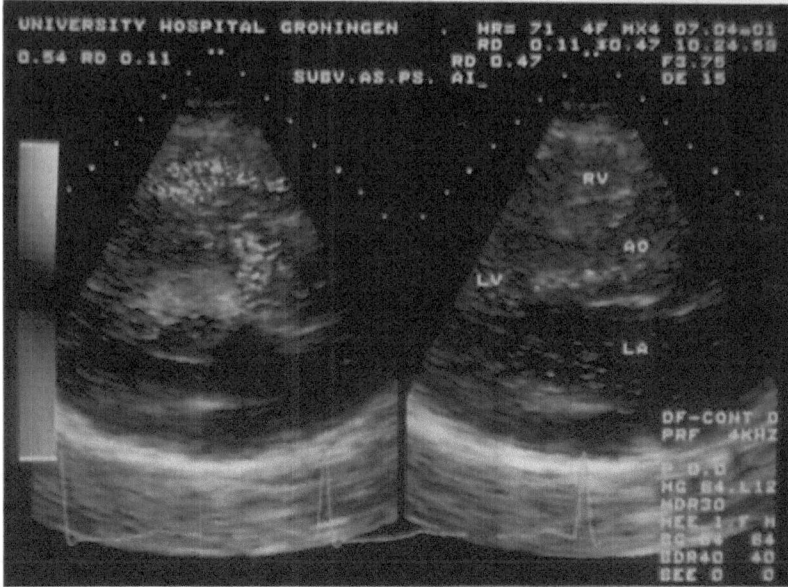

Fig. 8-38. Long axis view of a patient, suspected of having aortic stenosis and insufficiency. The turbulent colors in the LV outflow tract below the aortic valve indicate sub-valvular aortic stenosis. The diastolic frame (right) also shows aortic insufficiency (blue). However, turbulent colors are also recorded from the RV, showing also unsuspected sub-valvular pulmonic stenosis.

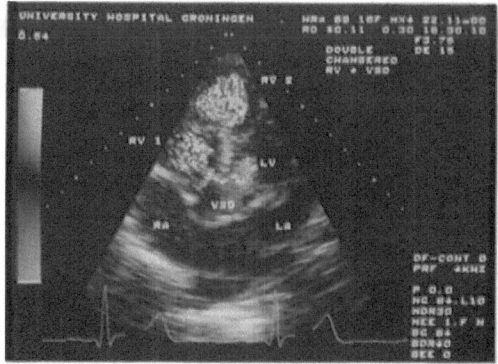

Fig. 8-39. Apical view during systole of an 18 year old boy with a double chambered RV and a VSD. A blue color with aliasing in the LV shows a flow from LV through the VSD. Turbulent colors just above the tricuspid valve (RV1) are abnormal and caused by the VSD. A 'septation' is found in the RV, with obstruction, also causing turbulent colors in RV2.

localization of an obstruction: unsuspected mid-ventricular obstructions or sub-valvular pulmonic stenosis have been found, simply by the presence of turbulent colors in the RV (Fig. 8-38).

In double chambered RV or (sub)valvular pulmonic stenosis, a VSD may also be present. For these combinations, color Doppler is very helpful in finding the correct diagnosis (Fig. 8-39).

Pressure measurements

Peak pressures in the RV can be calculated reliably with combined color Doppler and CW Doppler. In the absence of (sub)valvular pulmonic obstruction, this is also the peak pressure in the pulmonary artery.

For this measurement, tricuspid insufficiency has to be present. This is almost always the case in pulmonary hypertension (> 35 mm Hg peak pressure). The systolic blood velocity across the tricuspid valve is measured from the CW Doppler recording. To avoid under-estimation, the angle between the CW line and the direction of flow (as established with color Doppler) should be included in the calculation (Fig. 8-40).

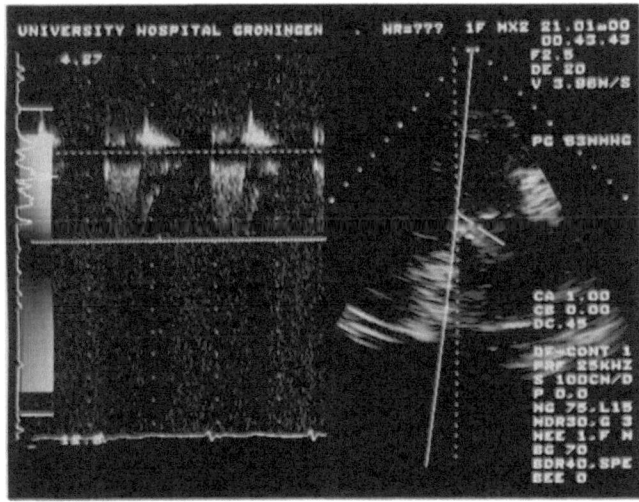

Fig. 8-40. Calculation of the flow velocity across the tricuspid valve with correction for the angle. The short axis aortic view was used as no colors could be detected from the apex. The blue color indicates flow from the RV (above) to the RA. The flow velocity, corrected for the angle results in a RV peak pressure of 63 mm Hg. Without angle correction this would have been 13 mm Hg. It should be noted that this angle is one of the largest found in our clinic and that it took much time to establish it as well as possible. At cardiac catheterization -one hour later- the peak pressure value was confirmed.

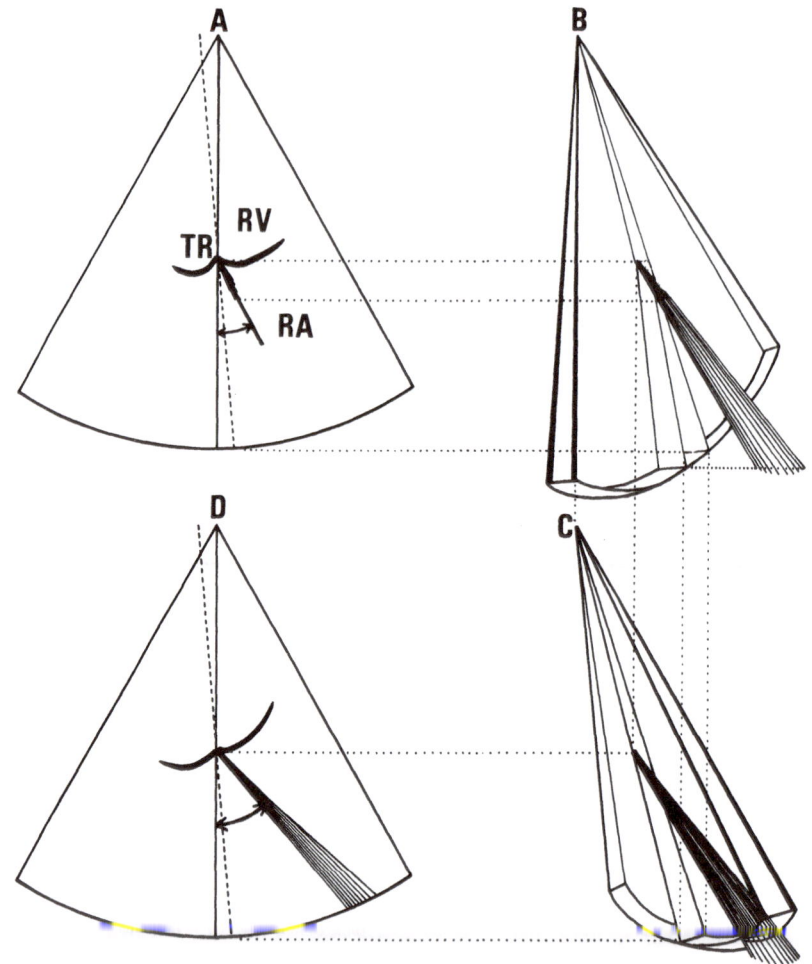

Fig. 8-41. Illustration of a cause of under-estimation of the angle. If the recorded color flow is short (A), there may be an angle between the sectorplane and the direction of flow (B). If the transducer is rotated (C), a longer color beam is recorded with a larger angle (D).

Often the best transducer position for calculating the angle is the short axis aortic view. Because of a shorter distance from the transducer, colors are better than from the apical view.

Establishing the angle can be rather time-consuming, especially if large angles are found. Small angles of less than 15° are unimportant. For large angles, the correction factor also becomes very large (Fig. 6-9). With this in mind, two conditions are important.

Firstly, the color flow should be as long as possible. With the point of leakage in the middle of the sector, the transducer should be rotated around its

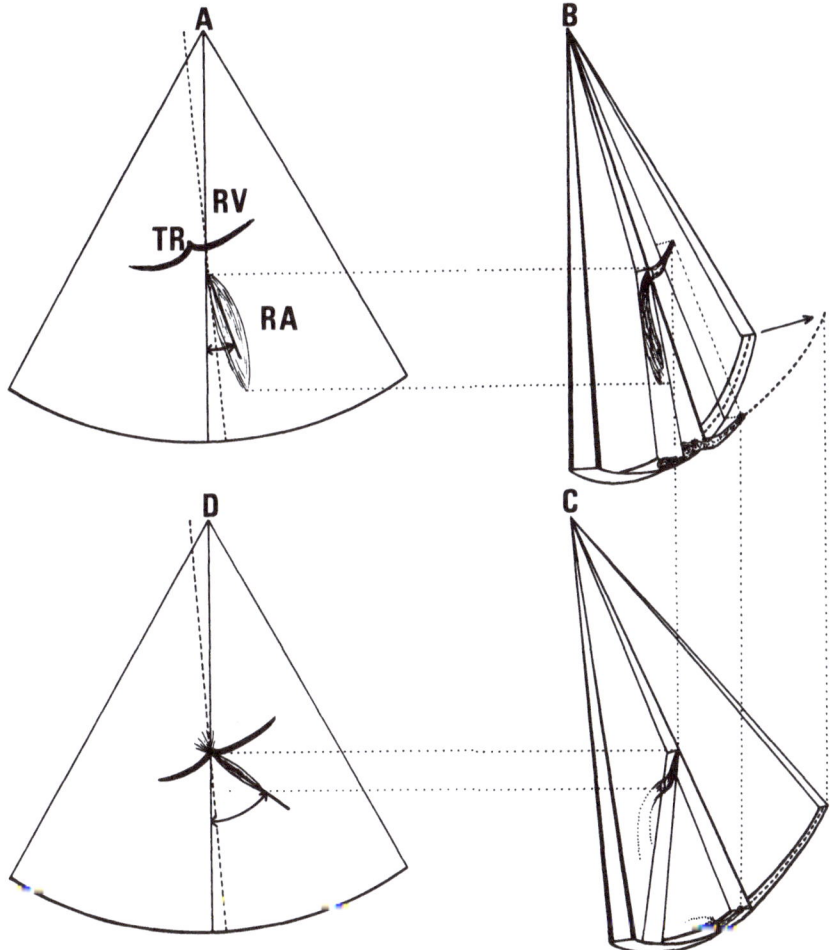

Fig. 8-42. Illustration of a cause of under-estimation of the angle. If the color flow direction should be curved and does not originate from the valve (A) the sectorplane should be moved to the right in this example (B) to detect the direction of flow immediately below the tricuspid valve. Then, with this point in the middle of the sector, the transducer is rotated around its long axis to make the color flow as long as possible, in the example clockwise ((B-C). This results in the correct angle (D).

long axis in order to make the angle as large as possible (Fig. 8-41).

This is to include a possible angle between the direction of flow and the sectorplane. The CW line is than positioned through the tricuspid valve and the flow velocity, corrected for the angle, is measured.

Secondly, the color flow should originate from the valve itself; if not, the angle can be under-estimated if the flow direction is curved (Fig. 8-42).

In other words: the color should originate from the ostium, this point has to be positioned in the middle of the sector and the transducer should be rotated then around its long axis to obtain the largest angle.

Peak pressures are easily obtained from CW recordings. With the simplified Bernoulli formula the flow velocity is converted into a pressure difference. As the pressure difference is obtained between RV and RA, the RA pressure should theoretically be included in the calculation to obtain the exact RV peak pressure. However, this pressure is usually low or not important compared to the increased RV pressure; it can be deleted and is not really helpful in clinical decision making.

(The method of roughly estimating the RA pressure is discussed in Chapter 8, under 'RA and IVC').

Pulmonary flow parameters can also be used to predict the presence of pulmonary hypertension. The time required to achieve the peak pulmonary flow velocity (acceleration time), and the ratio of acceleration time to RV ejection time can be measured directly from the pulmonary flow velocity curve. They have been shown to be inversely related to the pulmonary artery pressure. The acceleration time varies with heart rate and shortens with higher pulmonary artery pressures. Also, slight changes in sample volume position may significantly alter the shape of the flow velocity curve.

LEFT ATRIUM

The normal left atrium

Transducer positions

The LA can be evaluated from the parasternal, apical and subcostal region. The cranial wall of the LA can sometimes be evaluated from the suprasternal position, which is useful for visualizing contractions of the LA wall. It is found just below the right pulmonary artery. Far the best transducer position is obtained with TEE as the esophagus is located against the posterior wall of the LA.

Size and measurements

The normal LA is almost always ovally shaped. If enlarged, the shape often tends to be circular. The shape of the LA is easily changed as the pressure is usually low. So, it is advisable to make measurements from several directions

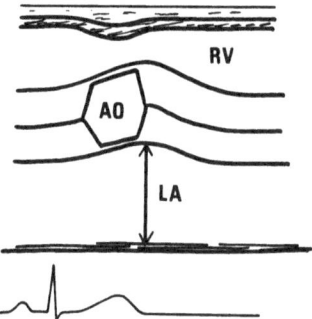

Fig. 8-43. Diagram illustrating the method of measurement of the LA diameter from the parasternal view. The measurement is made at the end of systole from the posterior wall of the aorta to the wall of the LA.

in order to obtain an impression of the volume. The antero-posterior diameter from the long axis view is obtained by positioning the M-line through the aortic valve, perpendicular to the aortic root. The LA diameter is the greatest distance between the posterior wall of the aorta and the posterior wall of the LA. This is at end-systole (Fig. 8-43). It is sometimes difficult to determine the posterior LA wall from this direction. This may be caused by side lobes, which can be excluded by rotating the transducer around its long axis.

A second diameter is obtained from the apical view, from the mitral leaflets to the cranial wall of the left atrium at end-systole (Fig. 8-44).

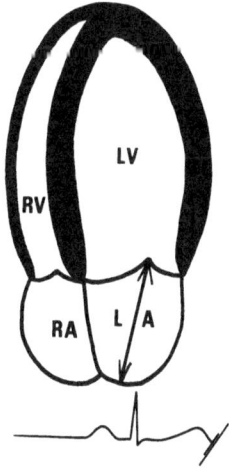

Fig. 8-44. Diagram illustrating the method of measurement of the LA diameter from the apical view. The measurement is made at the end of systole from the mitral leaflets to the cranial wall of the LA.

At least both dimensions should be mentioned in the report in order to give an impression of the volume. From the apical measurement no normal values are known; we use the values mentioned below.

Normal LA dimension from the long axis view 19-37 mm, mean 29 mm.
Normal LA dimension from the apical view 45-60 mm.

The abnormal left atrium

Function

From the flow velocities across the mitral valve, the mechanical activity of the LA can be visualized as the a-wave. The P-waves on the ECG, representing depolarisation of the atria, are not always followed by a clear mechanical activity.

In increased LVEDP, the E/A ratio from the mitral Doppler signal is less than 1,1.

Enlargement

The problems in the measurement of the LA make it questionable if minor enlargements can be detected reliably. Accurate measurements from at least two directions are at least necessary to obtain an impression of the LA volume (Fig. 8-58).

Enlargement of the LA is caused by volume and/or pressure overload and in long standing atrial fibrillation. Causes of volume overload are mitral insufficiency and VSD. Pressure overload is caused by mitral stenosis, increased LVEDP and masses in the LA, obstructing the mitral valve.

In pressure overload the inter-atrial septum bends outward towards the RA, unless the pressure in the RA is also increased. This sign, however, can be helpful in determining which pressure is higher: that from the RA or that from the LA.

Occasionally, a giant LA can be found without signs of pressure- or volume overload.

Contents

Thrombus masses, myxomas and malignancies can be found in the LA. They are discussed in Chapter 8, in the section 'tumors of the heart'.

A rare condition is the cor triatriatum. It is a congenital abnormality in which a membrane is found in the LA. Sometimes such a membrane causes

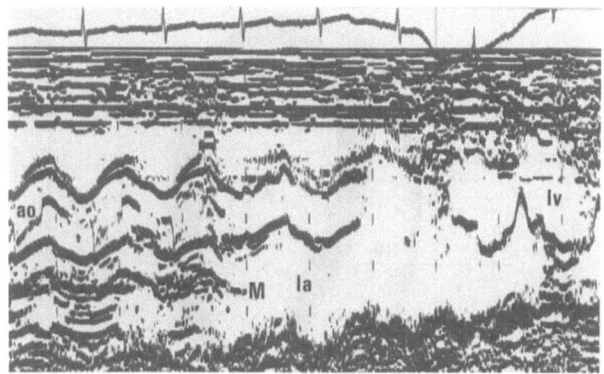

Fig 8-45. Left parasternal M-mode sweep of a cor triatriatum. Behind the aorta in the LA, a membrane (M) shows the presence of a cor triatriatrum.

obstruction between the cranial part of the LA and the LV (Fig. 8-45). The physical findings are the same as are found in mitral stenosis.

RIGHT ATRIUM and INFERIOR VENA CAVA

The normal right atrium

Transducer positions, size and measurements

The RA can be evaluated from the parasternal short axis aortic view, from the subcostal view, from the apical view (Fig. 8-46) and with TEE. Occasionally, evaluation from the right parasternal region is possible. For measurement of the size of the RA, the apical position is most suitable. The following can be taken as a normal value.

Normal RA dimension from the apical view < 55 mm.

Contents

Usually the RA is echo-empty but various structures can be found in a normal RA. Filamentous echoes can be present near the inter-atrial septum, representing residual tissue, the Chiari network (Fig. 8-47, 8-48). This is not considered to be an abnormality. A Chiari network has to be differentiated from a part of the inter-atrial septum in case of an ASD. Differentiation is possible with auscultation and/or TEE. Occasionally, these filamentous echoes may be confused with thin, also moving echoes that originate from an

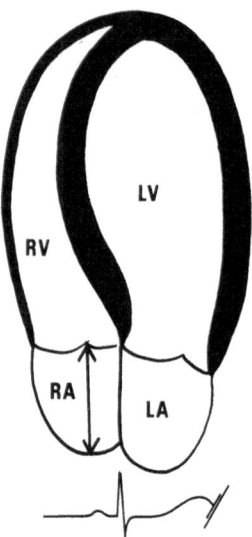

Fig. 8-46. Schematic illustration of a method of measurement of the RA.

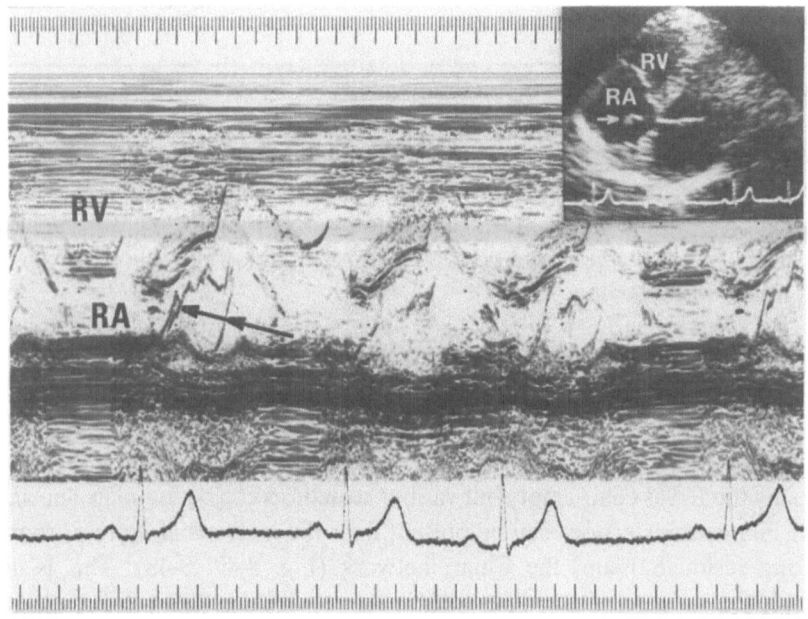

Fig. 8-47. Recording of a Chiari network (arrows) from the apical view. A quick motion of thin structures below the tricuspid valve is typical.

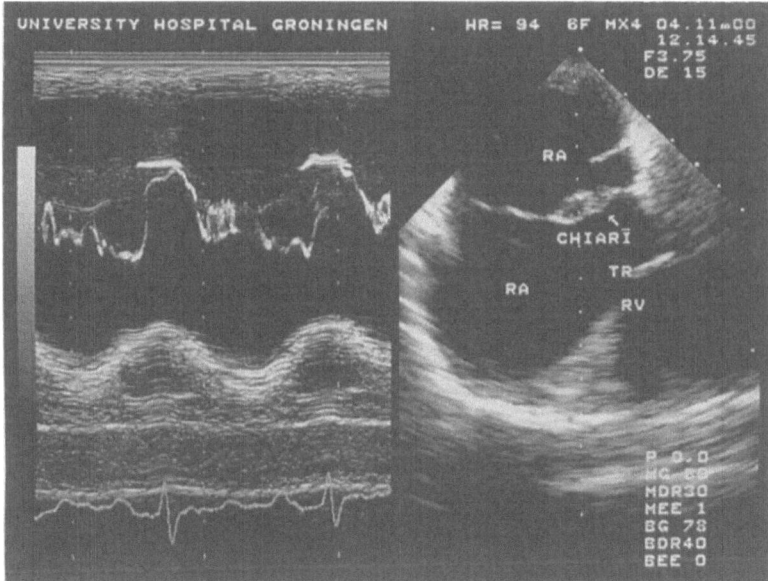

Fig. 8-48. A Chiari network from the TEE position. Long filaments are recorded in a rather large RA.

'echo-translucent' RA myxoma. Differentiation between both is possible with color Doppler and also with TEE.

The abnormal right atrium

Enlargement

Volume overload is the most common cause for RA enlargement. Causes may be tricuspid insufficiency, ASD and abnormal venous drainage. Occasionally, a shunt between the aorta and the RA causes volume overload.

The RA can also be enlarged by pressure overload when the RVEDP is increased as in pulmonary hypertension. Other causes are obstruction of the tricuspid valve by a stenosis or a tumor.

In pressure overload the inter-atrial septum bends out towards the LA, unless the pressure in the LA is also increased. This sign, however, can be helpful in determining which pressure is higher: that from the RA or that from the LA.

Another common cause for RA enlargement without pressure or volume overload is long standing atrial fibrillation.

Contents

Abnormal echo masses can be found in the RA, caused by thrombi or malignant and benign masses. This is discussed in Chapter 8, the section on tumors.

The inferior vena cava

With echocardiography, the IVC is sometimes confused with the abdominal aorta. They are differentiated by their relative positions and by the aspect of their walls. The IVC is on the right side of the abdominal aorta. The abdominal aorta has the same dimension throughout the picture, whereas the IVC usually becomes broader towards the RA. Echogenic parallel vessels are always seen from the aorta. Hepatic veins are helpful in identifying the IVC (Fig. 8-49). Systolic widening of an abdominal vessel is not specific to the aorta as it can also be seen from the IVC in the presence of tricuspid insufficiency.

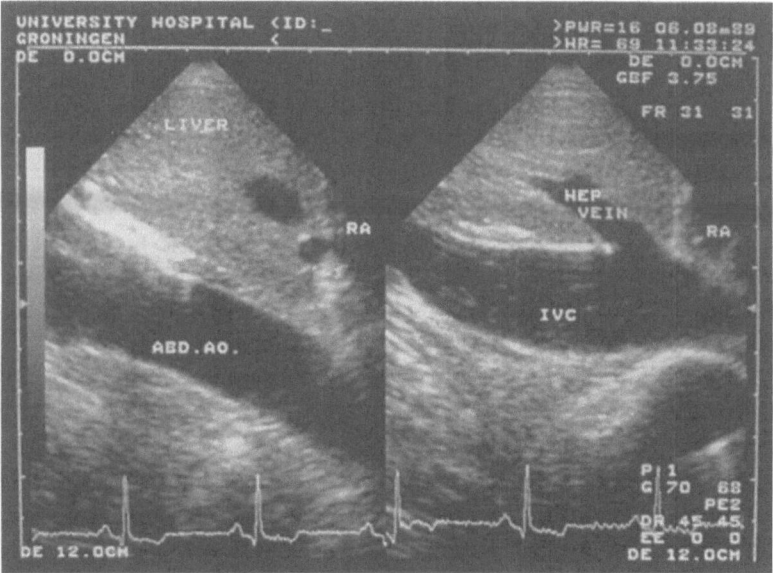

Fig. 8-49. The abdominal aorta and the IVC from the IVC view. The aorta has the same dimension throughout the picture, whereas the IVC becomes broader towards the RA. From the aorta echogenic parallel vessels are always recorded. Hepatic veins are helpful in identifying the IVC. Also, the IVC is on the right side of the abdominal aorta.

Diameters

There is a poor relationship between the diameters and pressures of the IVC. However, besides measurement of the central venous pressure as judged from the neck veins, a change in diameter of the IVC during respiration is helpful in differentiating between high and low pressures.

Normally, during inspiration, the lowered intra-thoracic pressure causes an increased flow towards the RA and because of this, the IVC collapses (Fig. 8-50).

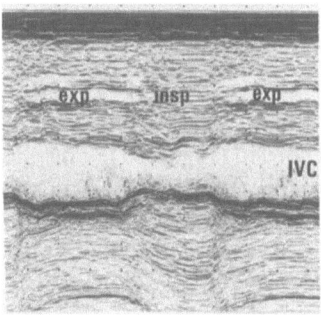

Fig. 8-50. M-mode recording at a paper speed of 25 mm/sec of the IVC. During expiration (exp) the diameter is 22 mm, during inspiration (insp) 10 mm. This collapse indicates that pressures in the IVC and in the RA and the RV end-diastolic pressure (if the tricuspid valve is normal) are normal.

In case of increased RA pressures, inspiration hardly influences this flow and hardly any or no collapse of the IVC is seen.

If the diameter of the IVC does not change during respiration, it is very likely that the pressure in the IVC is more than 7 mm Hg (normal pressure 2-4 mm Hg). The finding is important as, in the absence of significant tricuspid insufficiency, the pressure is the same as from the RVEDP. Indirectly, information is obtained about the diastolic function of the RV.

The behaviour of the IVC diameter during respiration only gives information about the pressure, not about the volume: in case of a normal collapse during inspiration, hemodynamically significant tricuspid insufficiency may be present with still low pressures. The severity of tricuspid insufficiency is best evaluated with a liver pulse recording.

Contents

Occasionally, the remnants of the Eustachian valve can be seen there, where the IVC enters the RA.

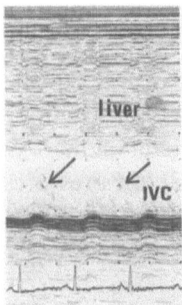

Fig. 8-51. M-mode recording during held expiration of the IVC. Spontaneous contrast is visible in the IVC (arrows) which has no pathologic meaning.

The IVC itself is echo-empty, but sometimes -in excellent conditions- spontaneous contrast can be recorded (Fig. 8-51). This has no meaning.

Echo masses can be found in the IVC, caused by a thrombus mass or by a Grawitz tumor, a malignant tumor from the kidney (Fig. 8-52). It may be difficult to differentiate between both, as the echo-density may be the same. If the IVC is locally dilated by an echo mass, a Grawitz tumor, which is a malignant tumor from the kidney, is likely to exist.

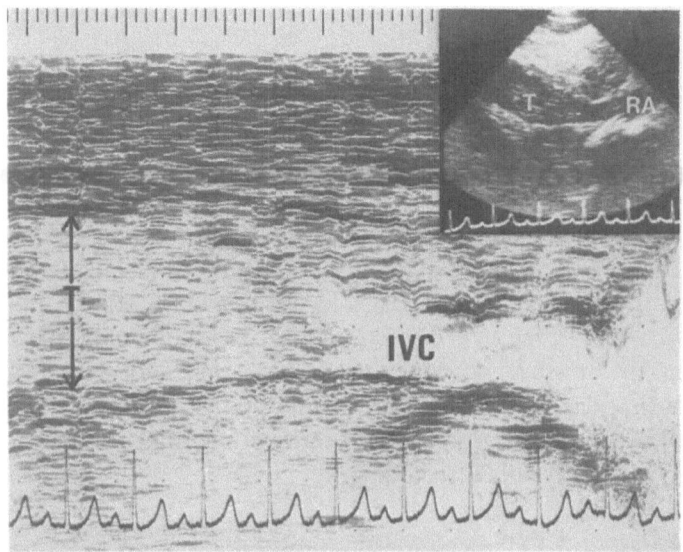

Fig. 8-52. Recording of abnormal echoes (T) in the IVC. As the IVC is dilated by an echo mass, it may be a malignant tumor, in this example a Grawitz tumor. The echo mass has to be differentiated from a thrombus mass, which is barely able to dilate the IVC.

AORTIC VALVE AND ROOT

The normal aortic valve and root

In normal conditions

The best position for imaging the whole aortic valve is the short axis aortic view. The three closure lines of the valve are visible then as an upside down Mercedes Benz symbol (Fig. 8-53). The aortic valve consists of three identical cusps. However, the left coronary cusp is sometimes smaller than the other cusps in a normal functioning valve (Fig. 8-54). The closure line between the

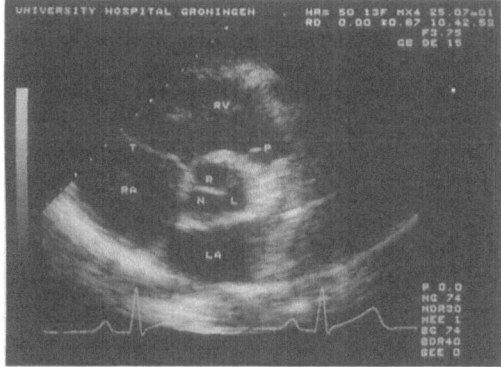

Fig. 8-53. Normal short axis aortic view. The aortic valve has three cusps, the right (R), the left (L) and the non-coronary cusp (N). T = tricuspid valve, P = pulmonic valve.

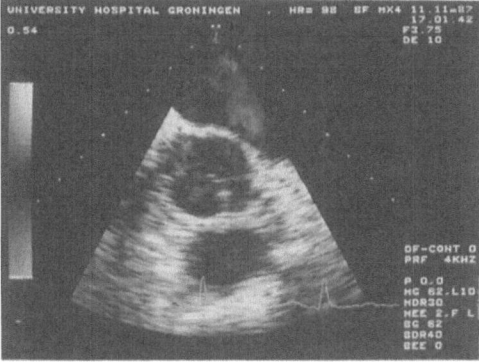

Fig. 8-54. The aortic valve from the TEE position. The left coronary cusp (on the right of the picture) is smaller than the other cusps. From this position, the non coronary cusp is the upper one.

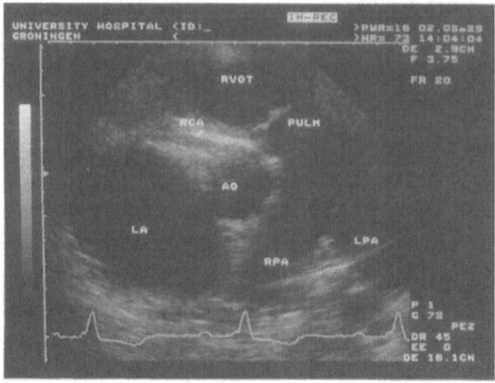

Fig. 8-55. Short axis view, just above the aortic valve, showing the first part of the right coronary artery (RCA). Also the right (RPA) and left pulmonary artery (LPA) are recorded.

left and the non-coronary cusp is often poorly visible as the ultrasound is parallel to this structure. Occasionally, the origin of the coronary vessels can be identified (Fig. 8-55).

M-mode recordings are made from the same position or from the parasternal long axis view. They can be used for the detection of small flutters and for the calculation of cusp separation and the ejection time. Normal cusp separation is 1.5-2.6 cm, mean 1.9 cm. This is, however, only a separation in one direction, which is not always representative for the whole aortic ostium. In the long axis view, the closure line of the valve is in the middle of the aortic root. An eccentric closure line may be caused by a congenital deformation, but can also be found in normal subjects. On the other hand, the closure line may be central in case of a bicuspid aortic valve. The normal aortic valve may show a physiological flutter at the leading edges of the cusps while valve separation is almost the same throughout systole (Fig. 8-56).

A coarse flutter can sometimes be recorded if a small cranial part of the IVS bulges out into the LV outflow tract. Often, this part of the IVS is slightly thickened in normal persons and also shows a good systolic thickening which discriminates the recording from HOCM.

The motion pattern of the aortic root roughly reflects the stroke volume: good excursions indicate a good stroke volume. The normal diameter of the aortic root is 2.0-3.7 cm, mean 2.7 cm.

In abnormal conditions

The M-mode recordings that can be obtained from the aortic valve – except for aortic stenosis – with the causes are schematically described in Fig. 8-57.

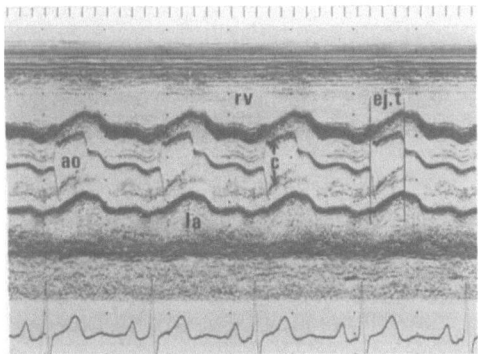

Fig. 8-56. M-mode recording of a normal aortic valve (ao). C indicates measurement of cusp separation. The ejection time (ej.t) is measured from the opening to the closure point of the valve and should be measured at a paper speed of at least 100 mm/sec. The good motion pattern of the aortic root reflects a good stroke volume.

In hypovolemia with a good quality LV, less blood passes the aortic valve during systole. The ejection time is shortened (Fig. 8-57F).

Another condition that can cause an abnormal M-mode recording of the aortic valve is impaired systolic LV function with a decreased stroke volume. Causes may be multiple myocardial infarctions and all types of cardiomyo-

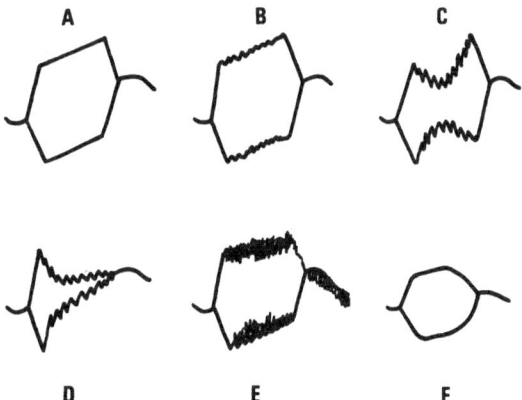

Fig. 8-57. Possible M-mode recordings of the aortic valve (except for aortic stenosis and sclerosis).
A = normal valve without flutter: normal conditions; congenital aortic stenosis
B = normal valve with systolic flutter: normal conditions
C = systolic flutter + midsystolic tendency to close: HOCM; sub-valvular membranous stenosis; sub-valvular jet without obstruction
D = systolic flutter + early syst tendency to close: sub-valvular membranous stenosis; HOCM
E = diastolic flutter + systolic thickening of cusps: vegetations; rupture
F = poor cusp separation + early closure without flutter: DCM; poor LV function

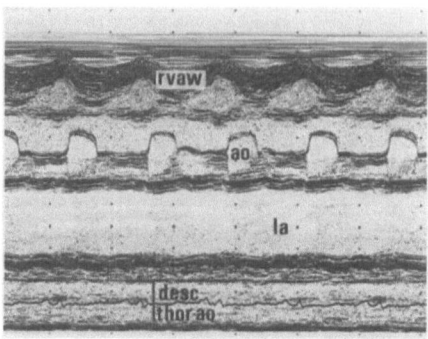

Fig. 8-58. M-mode recording of a normal aortic valve with poor excursions and an early tendency to close. The concomitant poor motion pattern of the aortic root indicates a low output LV. The RV anterior wall (rvaw) is thickened and very echogenic, so that amyloid is likely to be the cause. In the absence of mitral insufficiency the LA is usually enlarged by the increased LVEDP. On this recording however, the LA seems to be normal; this is caused by impression of the descending thoracic aorta (desc thor ao). From other views enlargement of the LA could easily be measured.

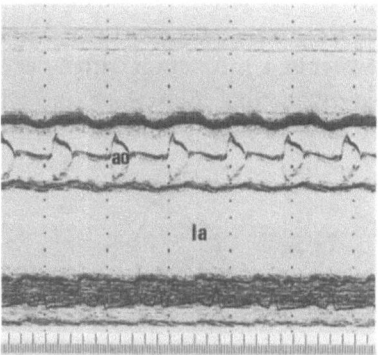

Fig. 8-59. M-mode recording of a normal aortic valve in DCM. The poor motion pattern of the aortic root indicates a small stroke volume. There is rather poor cusp separation with an immediate tendency to close with a very early closure of the valve. The LA is enlarged by the increased LVEDP and mitral insufficiency.

pathy. The aortic valve closes earlier, as the LV has no power to complete a normal systole. Also, in severe cases, the aortic valve does not open widely and has an early tendency to close, without a flutter (Fig. 8-58, 8-59). Simultaneously, diminshed excursions are found from the aortic root, caused by a small stroke volume.

Muscular sub-valvular obstruction causes a systolic jet in the LV outflow tract. The shape and the flow velocity of such a jet depend on the type, location and severity of the obstruction. A systolic jet in the LVOT may be caused by

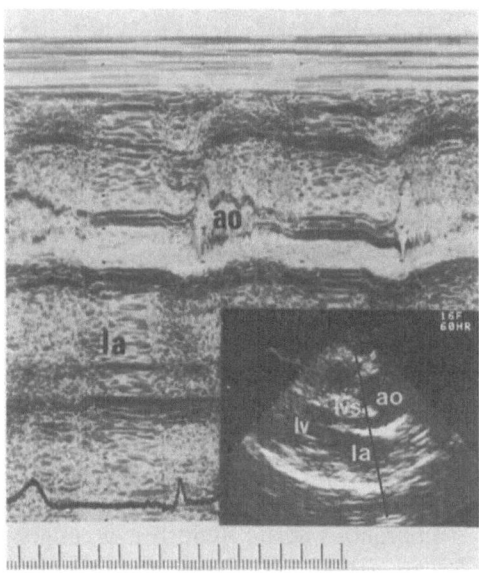

Fig. 8-60. Aortic valve (ao) with a normal initial opening and an early tendency to close with a coarse flutter on the leading edges of two cusps. The pattern is caused by some overriding of the aorta. There is no obstruction.

some overriding of the aorta (Fig. 8-60), by a sub-valvular membrane (sub-valvular membranous stenosis Fig. 8-61, 8-62) or by local thickening of the IVS (Chapter 8, HOCM, 'LV'). In all three conditions a coarse flutter of the aortic leaflets is recorded; also, after initial opening there is some tendency to close (Fig. 8-57C,D).

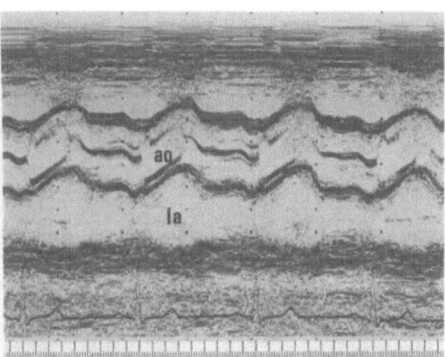

Fig. 8-61. Aortic valve (ao) with a normal opening of the lower cusp and an initial wide opening with a flutter and a tendency for the right coronary cusp to close. The pattern is caused by a membranous sub-valvular obstruction.

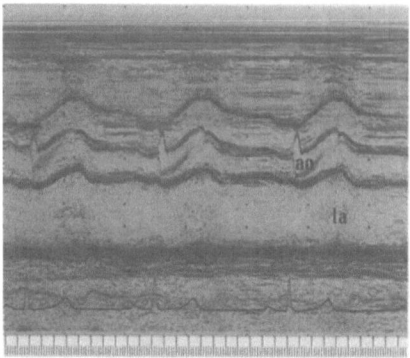

Fig. 8-62. The same type of recording as from Fig. 8-61. There is a greater tendency for the right coronary cusp to close and there is also a flutter on the other cusp.

A sub-valvular membranous aortic stenosis is a congenital disorder. The findings at physical examination and the symptoms depend on the severity of the obstruction and are the same as for aortic stenosis. A membrane is found attached to the IVS close to the aortic valve. This membrane causes obstruction of the LV outflow tract. From the parasternal long axis view, it is sometimes, but not always visible: the membrane is often smooth and, in this view, in line with the ultrasound beams. So, the echoes are sometimes clear (Fig. 8-63) but often poorly or not visible.

Better visualization can be expected from the apical view, when the ultrasound hits the membrane perpendicularly. Color Doppler is excellent for exact localization of the obstruction (Fig. 8-38, 8-64). With CW the pressure differ-

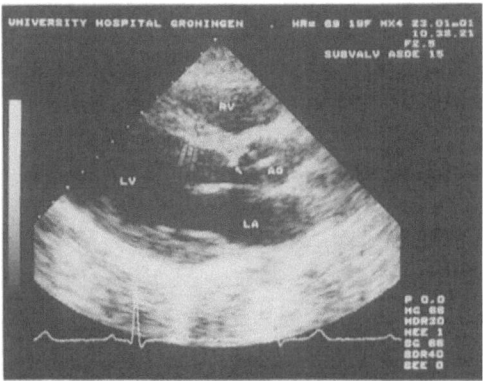

Fig. 8-63. Long axis parasternal view. In the LVOT, just below the aortic valve, a membrane is visible (arrow).

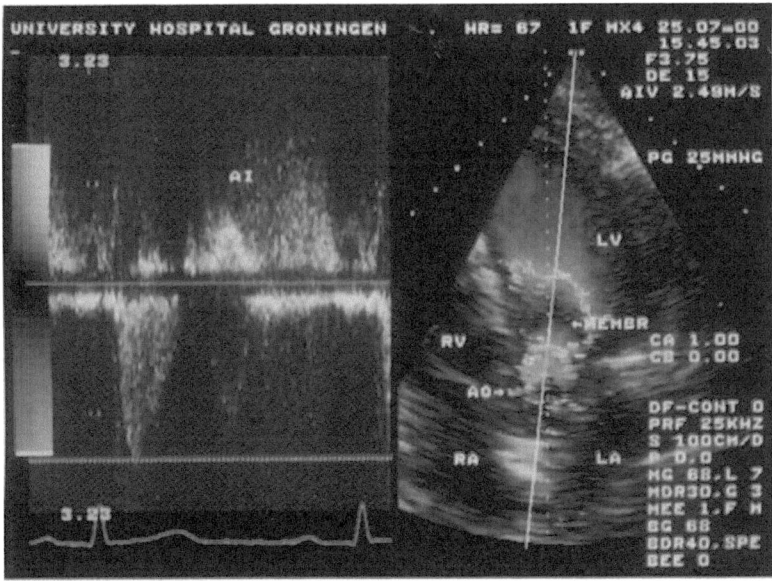

Fig. 8-64. Apical view in sub-valvular membranous stenosis. During systole the blue color with aliasing in the LVOT indicates flow velocity in the direction of the aorta. The black area in the LVOT is caused by the sub-valvular membrane (membr). Between membrane and aortic valve (ao) turbulent colors indicate a sub-valvular obstruction. The pressure difference across the membrane is 25 mm Hg at a heart rate of 67 b/min. This number is influenced by concomitant aortic insufficiency (AI).

ence across the membrane can be established from the apical view. In severe sub-valvular membranous stenosis a diffusely thickened LV wall is found with a good motion pattern.

To be investigated in sub-valvular aortic stenosis
echocardiography:
– location of the membrane (parasternal and apical views)
– coarse flutter on the M-mode recording of the aortic valve; a tendency to close (long axis view)
– LV wall thickness (long axis view)
– LV dimensions (long axis view)
– LA dimensions (long axis and apical view)
Doppler:
– pressure difference across the membrane together with heart rate during measurement
color Doppler:
– location of the obstruction (apical view)

124

pulse recording:
– a/H ratio (ACG)

The abnormal aortic valve and root

Congenital abnormalities

Instead of three equally large cusps, the aortic valve may consist of two or four cusps. The number and shape of the cusps can often be detected from the short axis aortic view. Often in the presence of two cusps (bicuspid valve) under-development or absence of the left coronary cusp is found and cusp separation is less wide than with three cusps (Fig. 8-65). Aortic stenosis however, is not necessarily present in this condition.

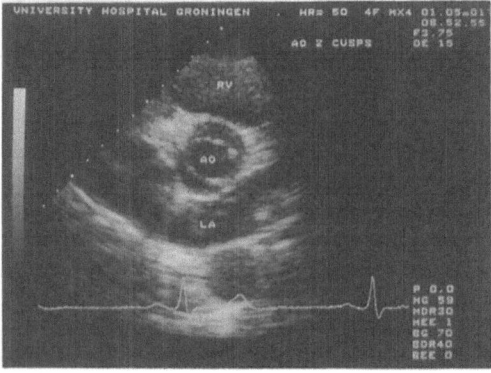

Fig. 8-65. Systolic short axis aortic view of a bicuspid aortic valve. The cusp separation is less wide than from a tricuspid aortic valve.

On the M-mode recording, the closure line of the valve may be eccentric. On the other hand, an eccentric closure line does not necessarily imply a bicuspid valve: it can also be found in normal aortic valves.

If the aortic valve is not screened carefully, a congenital aortic stenosis can be missed with echocardiography. The cusps are still smooth and often (especially from the long axis view) only the closure line is visible during diastole. During systole the basal parts of such 'dome-shaped' valves cause a falsely wide cusp separation. The ostium of the stenotic valve is not recorded then as it is in line with the ultrasound beams (Fig. 8-66).

To be investigated in congenital deformation of the aortic valve *echocardiography:*
– number and shape of cusps (short axis aortic view)

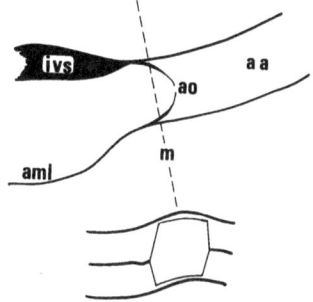

Fig. 8-66. Schematic representation of a possible under-estimation of congenital aortic stenosis. During systole, the dome-shaped aortic valve reflects ultrasound well from the base of the cusps. Poor or no echoes are recorded from the area of the aortic ostium (ao) where the ultrasound is (almost) parallel to the smooth cusps. An M-line (m) through the base of the valve will show good cusp separation on the M-mode recording in the presence of a possibly severe aortic stenosis. aa = ascending aorta.

- calcifications
- LV wall thickness (long axis view)
- LV dimensions (long axis view)
- LA dimensions (long axis and apical view)

CW Doppler:
- pressure difference (audio signal) across the valve together with heart rate during measurement (apical view). Quality of the CW signal.

ACG:
- a/H ratio for estimating the LVEDP.

Aortic stenosis

Aortic stenosis results in a pressure load for the LV. Only 2% is congenital, the majority is degenerative or caused by rheumatic heart disease.

The complaints and the findings on physical examinanation depend on the severity of the stenosis. In significant aortic stenosis, the patient is dyspnoic and shows fatigue on physical exertion. Angina is possible, caused by the increased oxygen demands of the LV with increased LVEDP. Fainting at rest or during physical exertion are serious symptoms as are rhythm disturbances.

On physical examination thrills may be palpable at the third intercostal space on the left side of the sternum, in the suprasternal notch, at the carotid arteries and/or at the apex (Fig. 8-74). The apex is accentuated and not displaced as long as there is no LV dilatation. The peripheral pulsations are weak.

In aortic stenosis leaflet separation is diminished on the M-mode recording

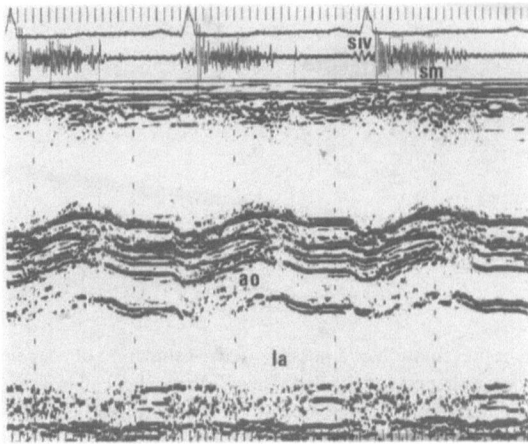

Fig. 8-67. Left parasternal M-mode recording of calcified aortic stenosis. It indicates the possible existence of aortic stenosis but cannot be proved: cusp separation is not always a reliable parameter for the presence and severity of aortic stenosis, it is also often barely measurable. In this recording, calcifications of the aortic valve prevent such measurements. The phonocardiogram shows a mid-late-systolic murmur (sm) and a fourth heart sound (SIV). Both indicate the existance of significant aortic stenosis. ao = aorta.

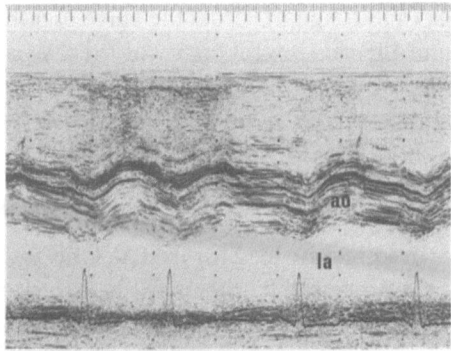

Fig. 8-68. Left parasternal M-mode recording of calcified aortic stenosis. It is not possible to even estimate the severity, since calcifications prevent any measurement. ao = aorta.

(Fig. 8-67, 8-68). On the other hand, the presence of aortic stenosis is sometimes poorly indicated by diminished leaflet separation. There is also a poor correlation between the measured cusp separation and the measured pressure difference across the valve.

Aortic stenosis may be absent in abnormal looking valves, but can also be surprisingly severe. One of the causes is that the aortic ostium is hardly ever circular shaped: leaflet separation, visualized from one direction does not necessarily reflect the ostium area. Another cause is the presence of calcifications which prevent exact visualization and determination of the size of the ostium.

Significant aortic stenosis causes thickening of the LV wall with normal LV diameters (Fig. 8-69, 8-70). Widening of the aortic root can be found but is more often seen in aortic insufficiency.

In very severe aortic stenosis a thickened LV wall is found, together with a poor motion pattern (Fig. 8-71). This gives the impression of an impaired LV function, but is only caused by the severe stenosis.

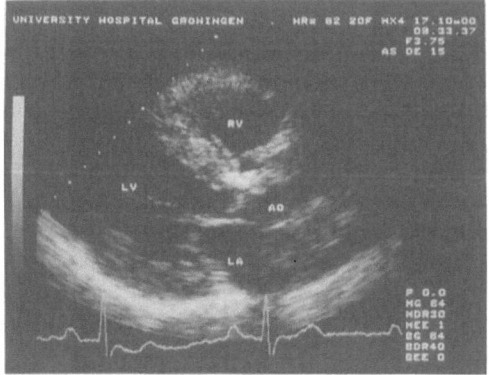

Fig. 8-69. Long axis view of aortic stenosis. The aortic valve is thickened with dense echoes, suggesting calcification. The LV is thick-walled and barely enlarged.

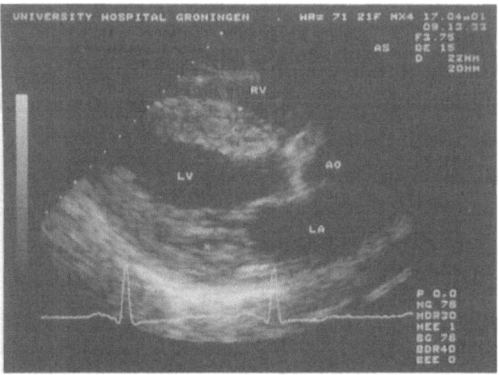

Fig. 8-70. Long axis view of severe aortic stenosis. The LV wall is strongly thickened (22,20 mm) and has a good motion pattern, suggesting hypertrophy. Dense echoes are visible from the closed aortic valve (ao).

128

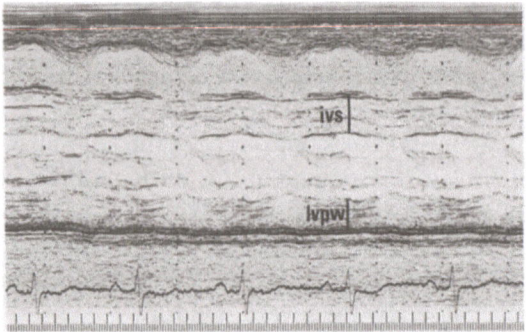

Fig. 8-71. Left parasternal M-mode recording of severe aortic stenosis. Both IVS and LVPW are greatly thickened. The poor motion pattern of the LV could be caused by a poor quality myocardium, but in this patient is caused by severe aortic stenosis. In fact, a combination of both possibilities cannot be excluded.

In elderly people fibrosis and calcification (sclerosis) of the aortic leaflets can be found without aortic stenosis. Diminished separation of thickened valves are recorded on M-mode. This condition can remain stable for many years. Sclerosis, however, can also change into a severe aortic stenosis within one year. If aortic sclerosis is found, echocardiographic controls should be performed regularly.

If the pressure difference across a stenotic aortic valve cannot be obtained, the murmur can be recorded together with the carotid pulse for calculating the Q to peak-of-murmur time and the ETI (Fig. 8-72, 8-73). The time, needed for the carotid pulse to reach half of its total deflection ($t^1/_2$Hcar) is lengthened.

If the Q-peak time is more than 190 ms, aortic stenosis may be present. If (in the presence of a normal LV function and in the absence of severe hypertension, significant mitral insufficiency or significant aortic insufficiency) the ETI is more than 420 ms (e.g. 430-480 ms), aortic stenosis may be significant. If $t^1/_2$ Hcar is 35 ms or more, aortic stenosis may be present. However, if abnormal, none of these parameters alone is a proof; it is only a good indication for aortic stenosis.

In LV failure the LVEDP is increased. For estimation of the LVEDP, the a/H ratio can be calculated from the ACG (Fig. 8-74).

The severity of aortic stenosis is best measured with CW from the apical view. Often, the suprasternal and supraclavicular positions can also be used. From the apical position, the CW beam can easily be aligned with the stenotic jet by listening to the audio signal. The instantaneous peak pressure difference across the aortic valve is calculated from the maximal flow velocity. At cardiac catheterization, a peak to peak pressure difference is measured: a non-physiological measurement that results in under-estimation of the severity of aortic

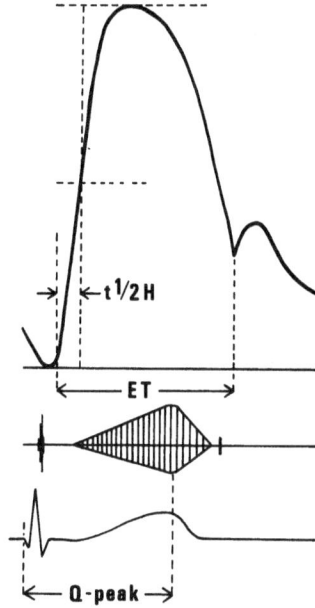

Fig. 8-72. Diagram of the measurements that can be made from the carotid pulse recording, the phonocardiogram and the ECG to evaluate aortic stenosis. $t^1/_2H$ = time, needed for the upstroke of the carotid pulse to reach half its maximum, ET = ejection time, Q-peak = time between the Q of the ECG and the peak of the systolic murmur.

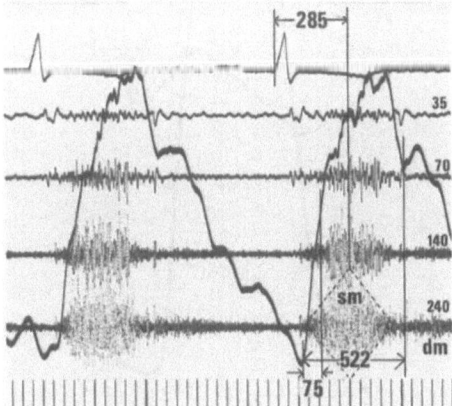

Fig. 8-73. Phonocardiogram on the third rib on the left with recording of the left carotid pulse in severe aortic stenosis. Both $t^1/_2H$ and ETI are lengthened, and a thrill is recorded on top of the pulse recording. The systolic murmur (sm) has a late maximum. A diastolic murmur (dm) indicates aortic insufficiency. Cut-off frequencies are 35, 70, 140 and 240 Hz.

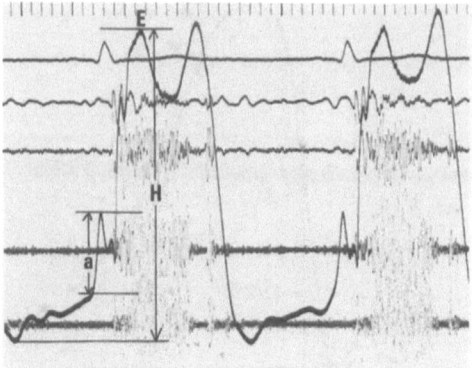

Fig. 8-74. Phonocardiogram on the third rib on the left with the apexcardiogram in aortic stenosis. A thrill is recorded during systole. The a-wave (a) is 28% of the total deflection as measured from the baseline to point E. This percentage indicates increased LVEDP, also about 28 mm Hg.

stenosis (Fig. 8-75). The more severe aortic stenosis is, the less important is the difference between both measurements. If the same methods are used, correlations with simultaneous measurements during cardiac catheterization are excellent. If comparing non-simultaneous measurements, one should also realize that pressure differences vary with heart rate, medication, sedation and other conditions.

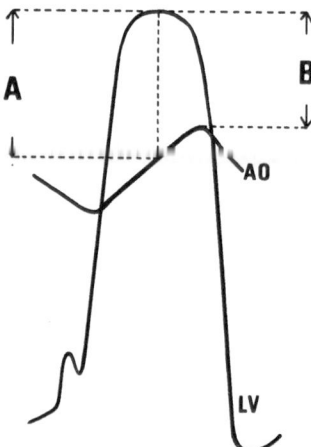

Fig. 8-75. Measurement of the peak pressure difference in aortic stenosis. The peak to peak pressure difference (B) is measured at cardiac catheterization. 'A' is the instantaneous peak pressure difference as measured with Doppler. If compared with Doppler, catheterization pressure measurements underestimate the severity of aortic stenosis. The less severe aortic stenosis is, the greater the difference between both measurements. LV = LV pressure recording, AO = aortic pressure recording.

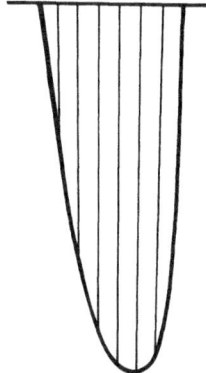

Fig. 8-76. Schematic CW signal of aortic stenosis as obtained from the apex. The mean pressure difference can be obtained by measuring the pressure differences at 5 points or more along the curve. The values obtained are averaged.

The mean gradient is calculated by measuring the peak flow velocities at 5 or more intervals along the flow velocity curve (Fig. 8-76). The peak pressure differences at these points are measured and averaged. The peak and mean pressure differences can directly be measured from the monitor by tracing the flow velocity curve (Fig. 8-77).

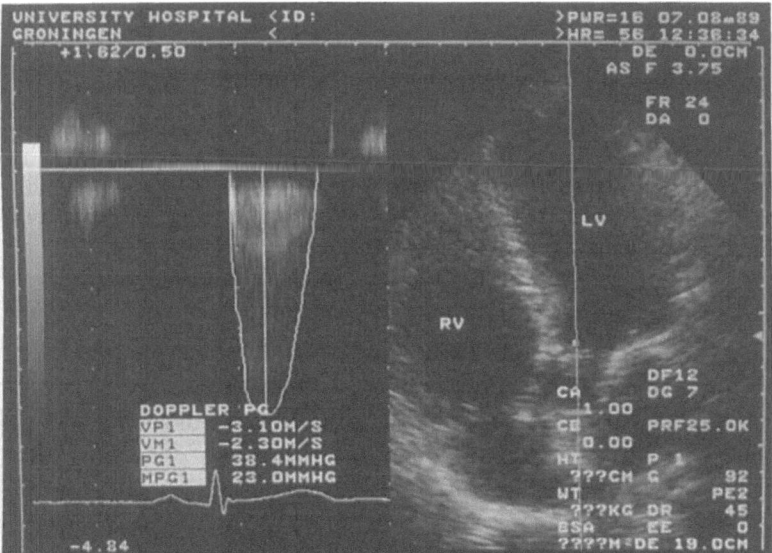

Fig. 8-77. Apical CW recording of aortic stenosis. A tracing of the flow velocity curve results in a peak pressure difference across the valve of 38 mm Hg and a mean pressure difference of 23 mm Hg at a heart rate of 56 b/min, which is a moderate aortic stenosis.

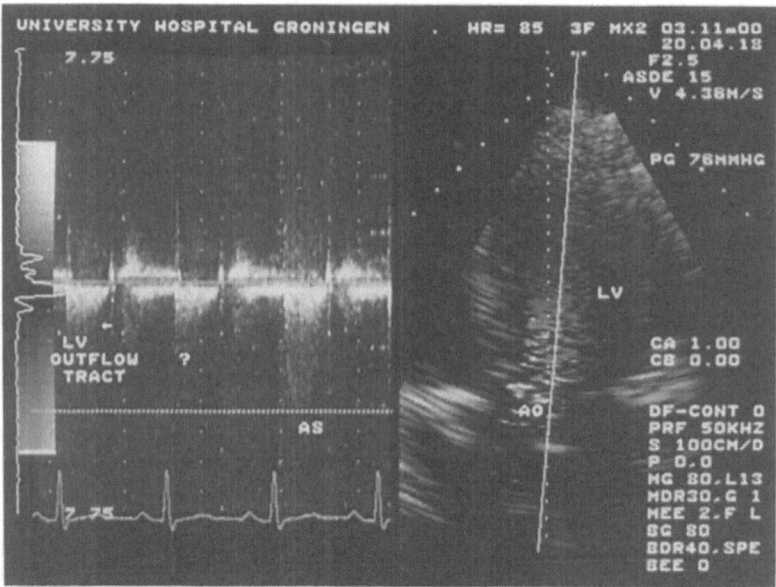

Fig. 8-78. Apical CW measurement of aortic stenosis. The first negative Doppler signal is caused by the LV outflow tract, the second one shows a larger amplitude of a weak signal that is clear in the third signal. From this third weak signal a peak pressure difference of 76 mm Hg at a heart rate of 85 b/min is measured (AS).

The mean pressure difference is a more sensitive measure of the severity of aortic stenosis as it less influenced by reduced cardiac output.

Under-estimation of the severity
Under-estimation of the severity of aortic stenosis is possible if the Doppler recording is not made correctly, if severe mitral insufficiency or coarctation of the aorta is also present and/or if the systolic LV function is impaired.

Instead of the flow velocity through the aortic ostium, the flow velocity in the LV outflow tract may be recorded (Fig. 8-78).

However, the audio signal from the outflow tract has not the characteristic high pitch of aortic stenosis. If, in suspected aortic stenosis, pressure differences of 10-20 mm Hg are found with CW Doppler from the apical view, care should be taken to determine whether the signal was obtained from the outflow tract or from the aortic ostium, especially if the signal has no sharp outline. Also, normal outflow tract CW signals have an early peak velocity. In aortic stenosis, the peak velocity is mid-to-late-systolic. Consequently, low pressure differences with a late-systolic CW peak velocity are caused by flow velocities of the outflow tract, but there is also aortic stenosis: further investigation is necessary to detect the flow velocity through the aortic ostium.

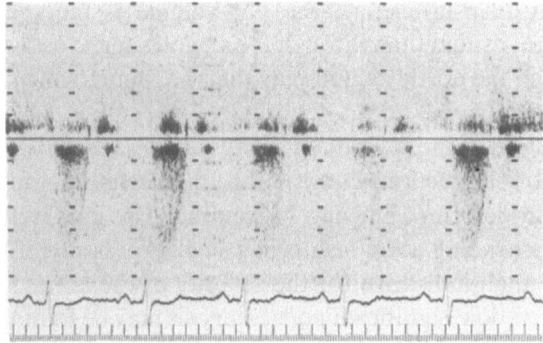

Fig. 8-79. Apical CW recording of aortic stenosis. The signal is weak and sometimes barely measurable. Respiration often makes the recording more difficult.

Theoretically, the problem could be solved with PD but the sample volume is far from the transducer and the velocities are high. This makes PD less suitable for measurement of flow velocities in aortic stenosis in the adult. However, color Doppler is helpful for the localization: the ostium is small and far away from the transducer and visualization with color is time-saving to locate the CW sound beam in the correct place.

Another source of under-estimation is a weak CW signal (Fig. 8-79). Also, the position of the aortic ostium with respect to the transducer changes easily with respiration. In this respect, the audio signal is most valuable in recognizing the correct signal. It should also be remembered that the CW gain setting must be as high as possible in order to detect weak signals (Fig. 8-80).

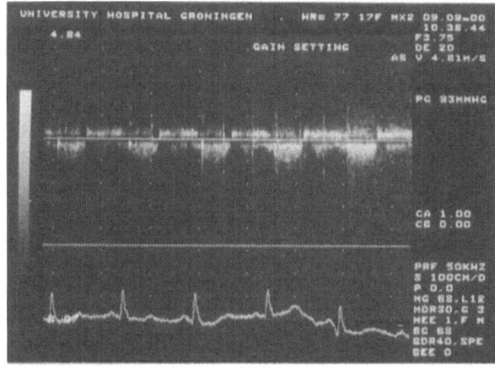

Fig. 8-80. Apical CW recording of aortic stenosis. A low gain setting (left) obscures the CW signal. With high gain settings, a weak signal shows a pressure difference of 93 mm Hg at a heart rate of 77 b/min.

In severe mitral insufficiency, the LV volume is more easily pumped through the mitral ostium than through the stenotic aortic ostium. Lower flow velocities through the aortic ostium may then be found, which are not representative of the severity of aortic stenosis.

Under-estimation of the severity of aortic stenosis with CW is also possible in the presence of obstructions in the aorta. In coarctation, the aortic valve is often congenitally deformed and may be stenotic. Also in coarctation, the high pressure in the ascending aorta results in a smaller pressure difference across the aortic valve than indicative for the severity of the aortic stenosis. After surgery for coarctation, significant aortic stenosis may be found that could not be detected before surgery. In this respect, the echocardiographic anatomy of the aortic valve should carefully be investigated.

Under-estimation of the severity of aortic stenosis is possible if cardiac output is reduced. Impairment of the LV function may be caused by the aortic stenosis itself or by myocardial infarction and cardiomyopathies. The peak pressure difference is not representative for the area of the aortic ostium. The mean pressure difference is more reliable.

Under-estimation is also possible if the angle between direction of flow and Doppler sound beam is not included in the calculation. From the apical view, however, the angle is usually too small to be significant. Also, visualization of the flow direction in the ascending aorta is hardly ever possible from the apical view: in many adults dense echoes from the aortic valve are found, preventing visualization of color behind the valve.

Over-estimation of the severity
The severity of aortic stenosis can be over-estimated with CW Doppler if aortic insufficiency is also present. In pure aortic insufficiency, pressure differences of 20-40 mm Hg can be found across the aortic valve (Fig. 8-81) in the presence of a definitely normal opening pattern of the valve cusps. Such measurements indicate correctly the pressure difference but can not be used for the calculation of the aortic ostium area.

Occasionally, very high flow velocities (indicating pressure differences of about 90 mm Hg) can be found in the absence of severe aortic stenosis. The CW signal from these flow velocities is always weak and difficult to detect and often obtained from the septal side of the ostium. Such pressure differences have also been found with Doppler during simultaneous cardiac catheterization; a CW pressure difference of 35 mm Hg easier to find with a better quality of the signal, which is then the same as measured with the catheter. The explanation of this difference is possibly the same as for false measurements from prosthetic valves.

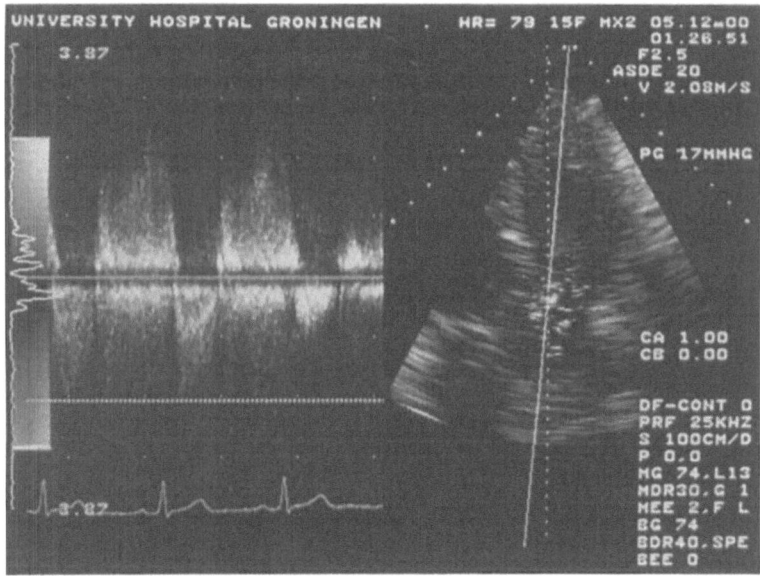

Fig. 8-81. Apical CW recording of aortic insufficiency. The systolic Doppler signal results in a pressure difference of 17 mm Hg across the aortic valve in the presence of a normal opening pattern of the cusps.

To be investigated in aortic stenosis
echocardiography:
– shape and number of cusps, intensity of the echoes from the valve (short axis aortic view, long axis view)
– LV wall thickness (long axis view)
– LV wall dimensions (long axis view)
Doppler:
– pressure difference (audio signal) through the ostium together with heart rate during measurement (apical view, suprasternal view). Quality and reliability of the CW signal. Peak and mean pressure differences.
color Doppler:
– localization of the aortic ostium, in order not to confuse the CW signal from the aortic ostium with that from the LV outflow tract (apical view)
TEE:
– sometimes helpful for further anatomic definition of the valve
pulse recording:
– a/H ratio for estimation of the LVEDP
– if the pressure difference can not be measured: Q-peak time, $t^1/_2$Hcar, ETI
If rhythm disturbances are seen during the examinations, they must be reported.

In the presence of aortic sclerosis and/or unsignificant aortic stenosis it is advisable to repeat measurements regularly. After the patient was examined for the first time, a second examination should be made after e.g. 6 months. If measurements are the same then, the intervals between the examinations can be lengthened.

Aortic insufficiency

Causes for aortic insufficiency are congenital deformation, inflammations, Marfan syndrome, and dissection of the aorta. Aortic insufficiency is not found in normal aortic valves.

Minor insufficiencies may be difficult to detect. It is not a threat to the LV function, but the diagnosis is important as aortic insufficiency is a well known cause for endocarditis and the patient should be warned. The diagnosis of a hemodynamically significant aortic insufficiency is often easy to make. Expressing the severity however, can be difficult.

Symptoms and physical findings depend on the severity. In severe insufficiency, the patient has dyspnea and fatigue on physical exertion. Also lightheadedness is common. In acute aortic insufficiency the patient is often aware of every heartbeat, caused by the larger stroke volume and the quick drop in pressure at end-systole.

At physical examination the apex is accentuated and often displaced to the left and downward. A diastolic murmur is heard in the third intercostal space at the left. Occasionally, a systolic thrill is palpable in the absence of aortic stenosis. In severe cases the head may bob with each heartbeat. Pulsations of the peripheral arteries are of the waterhammer type.

Direct features
With echocardiography, aortic insufficiency can often be suspected from the aspect of the valve (Fig. 8-82, 8-83, 8-84). Transducer positions for the evaluation of the valve are the long axis, short axis aortic, and occasionally the subcostal view. TEE can provide excellent pictures. If all three cusps are not equally large, aortic insufficiency may be present. Very often, some insufficiency is found in sclerotic valves. If caused by endocarditis, valve vegetations can be seen and/or valve rupture. The aspect of vegetations can be the same as from rupture: a small structure, attached to the closed aortic valve with a flutter during diastole and often also during systole. TEE can be helpful in the differentiation between the two. However, a pre-surgical differentiation is not always necessary.

CW Doppler. Aortic insufficiency is detected with CW Doppler by visible and audible signals. In this respect, the audio signal is often more conclusive,

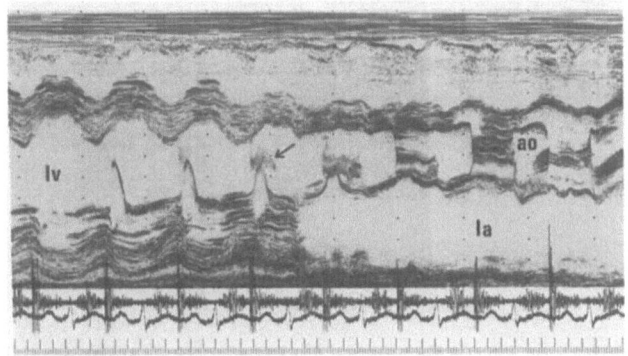

Fig. 8-82. Left parasternal long axis M-mode sweep. The LV dimensions are enlarged, there is a very good contraction pattern and LVPW thickness is normal. This is consistent with LV volume overload. Closure of the mitral valve is too early and is caused by increased LV diastolic pressure. The aortic valve opens widely and shows a mobile thickening of the cusps, indicative for valve vegetations. Part of the vegetations or part of a cusp hangs in the LV outflow tract during diastole (arrow).

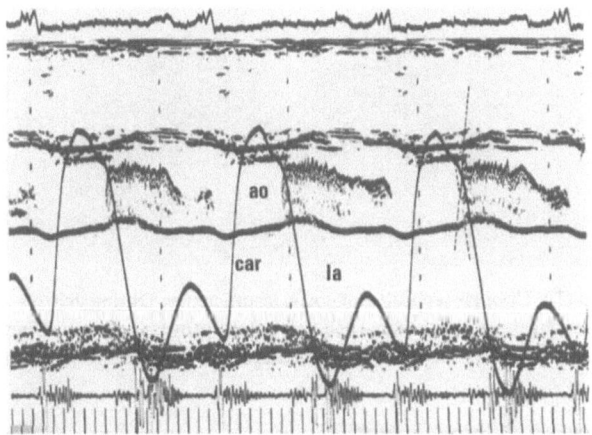

Fig. 8-83. Left parasternal M-mode recording of the aortic valve area with the carotid pulse recording. Only the right coronary cusp is recorded during systole. During diastole a fluttering structure, starting divergently, indicates valve rupture with vegetations. Because of severe aortic insufficiency the incisura of the carotid pulse recording is absent. car = carotid pulse recording.

especially in mild insufficiency. The apical view is usually the best view, as the flow is directed then towards the transducer. A positive signal starts with aortic closure with a down slope during diastole (Fig. 8-85). A steep down slope is suggestive for severe insufficiency, as pressures in the aorta and in the LV obviously equal fast.

138

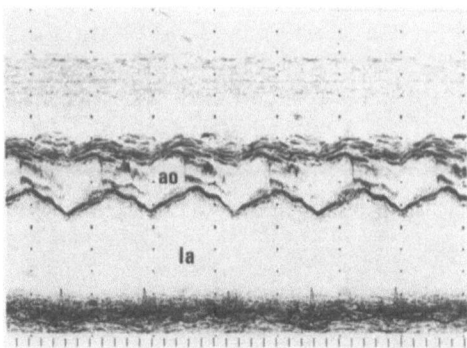

Fig. 8-84. Left parasternal M-mode recording, just below the aortic valve. Fluttering structures during diastole suggest vegetations and/or valve rupture. Both were confirmed at surgery.

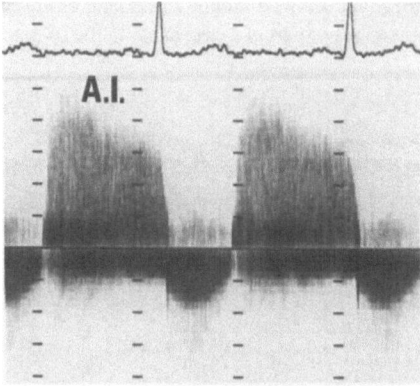

Fig. 8-85. Apical CW Doppler recording of aortic insufficiency. During diastole a positive signal, immediately following the negative signal of aortic inflow, proves aortic insufficiency. As shown in this recording, it is not always easy to obtain a measurable downslope. A.I. = aortic insufficiency.

In the presence of mitral insufficiency, the early closure of the mitral valve by severe aortic insufficiency may even cause a diastolic mitral insufficiency (Fig. 8-86).

The $t^{1}/_{2}p$ value, as used in calculating the severity of mitral stenosis, could also be applied to the CW signal of aortic insufficiency. However, correlations ranging from highly significant to rather poor with angiocardiography have been found. A $t^{1}/_{2}p$ value < 250 ms should indicate the presence of severe insufficiency.

Color Doppler. Aortic insufficiency can be visualized from various views with color Doppler: the short axis aortic, the long axis, the apical, the suprasternal view, occasionally from the subcostal view and from recordings of the femoral

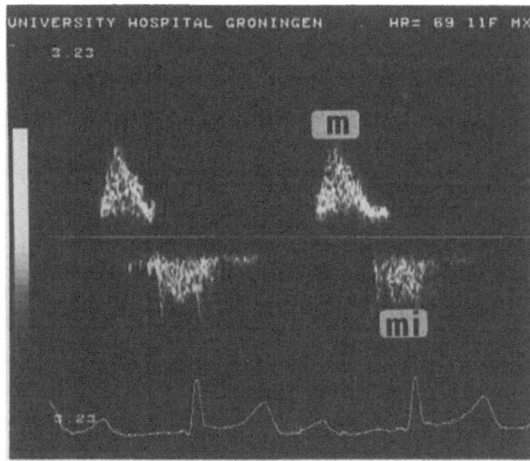

Fig. 8-86. Apical CW Doppler recording of the mitral flow velocity in the presence of severe aortic insufficiency. The quick rise in diastolic pressure, in combination with a first degree A-V block, cause a diastolic mitral insufficiency. m = mitral inflow, mi = mitral insufficiency.

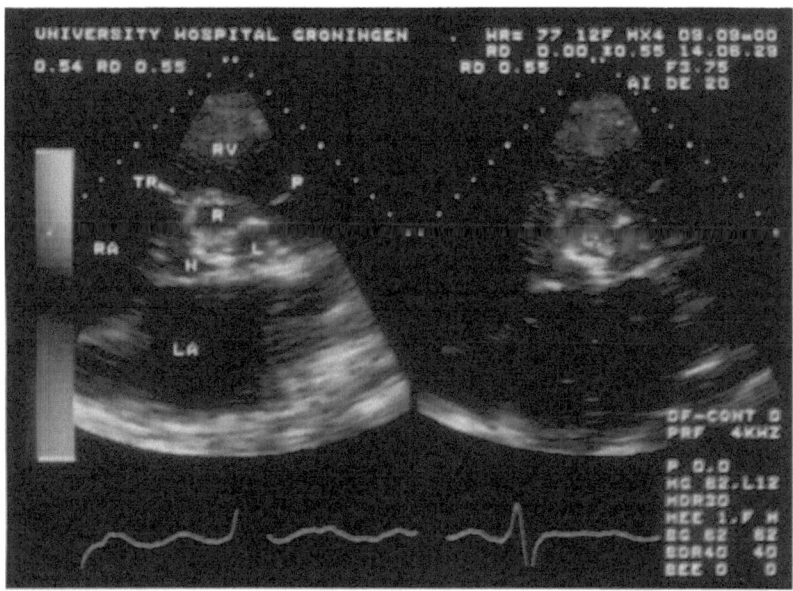

Fig. 8-87. Short axis aortic view of aortic insufficiency. Both frames are diastolic. On the left there seems to be a defect between the right (R) and non coronary cusp (N). Colors in that area in the right frame prove aortic insufficiency. L = left coronary cusp, TR = tricuspid valve, P = pulmonic valve.

140

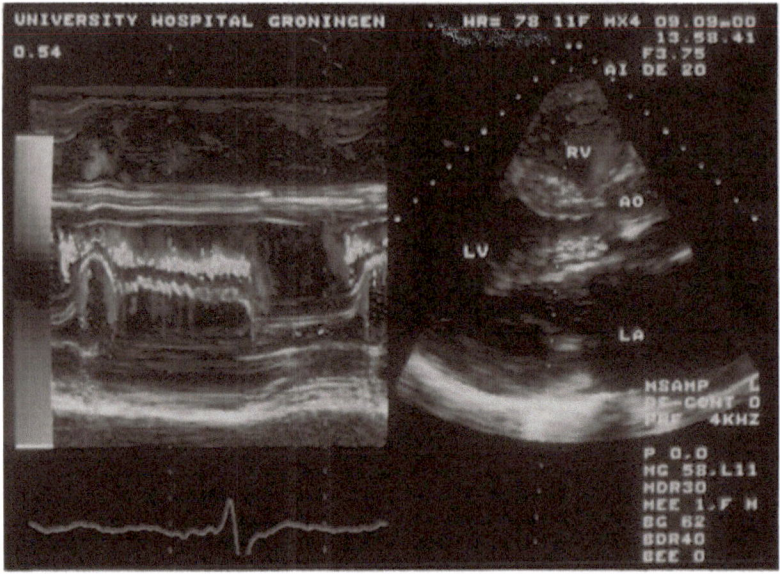

Fig. 8-88. Long axis view of aortic insufficiency. The diastolic sector frame shows a thickened aortic closure line and an enlarged LV. A turbulent flow with blue colors originates from the aortic valve and proves aortic insufficiency. On the M-mode recording the motion pattern of the LV is very poor, also taken into account that it should be extremely good, caused by the volume overload. It suggests myocardial failure. The turbulent colors are already visible before the mitral valve opens, which is the best proof of aortic insufficiency. The color flow strikes along the AML and causes a flutter of this leaflet.

artery and with TEE. Sometimes, minor insufficiencies can only be detected with one of all the views mentioned above.

From the short axis aortic view, no color is found during diastole in the normal valve. If colors are present, they prove aortic insufficiency, (Fig. 8-87). There is, however, a poor correlation between the color area measured from the diastolic phase of the short axis aortic view, and the severity of aortic insufficiency.

The long axis view can provide clear 'turbulent' colors from aortic insufficiency, surrounded by blue or red. The color depends on the direction of flow with respect to the transducer (Fig. 8-88).

The apical view is usually the best view for visualization of aortic insufficiency as the flow is directed then towards the transducer (Fig. 8-89). From this view, turbulent colors show the regurgitant flow. The red color on the right is caused by mitral inflow. Thus, timing is important to differentiate between aortic insufficiency and normal mitral inflow; with M-mode the flow from aortic insufficiency starts before the opening of the mitral valve (Fig. 8-88).

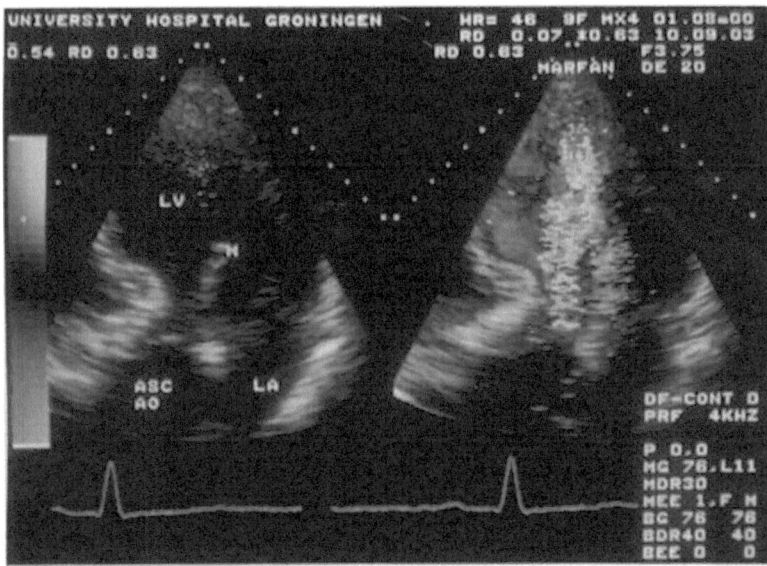

Fig. 8-89. Apical color Doppler recording of aortic insufficiency in Marfan. Both frames are diastolic. The left frame shows the AML (M) and the ascending aorta (ASC AO). The right frame is identical, but with color. Turbulent colors, originating from the aortic valve, indicate aortic insufficiency. The red color on the atrial side of the AML is caused by mitral inflow.

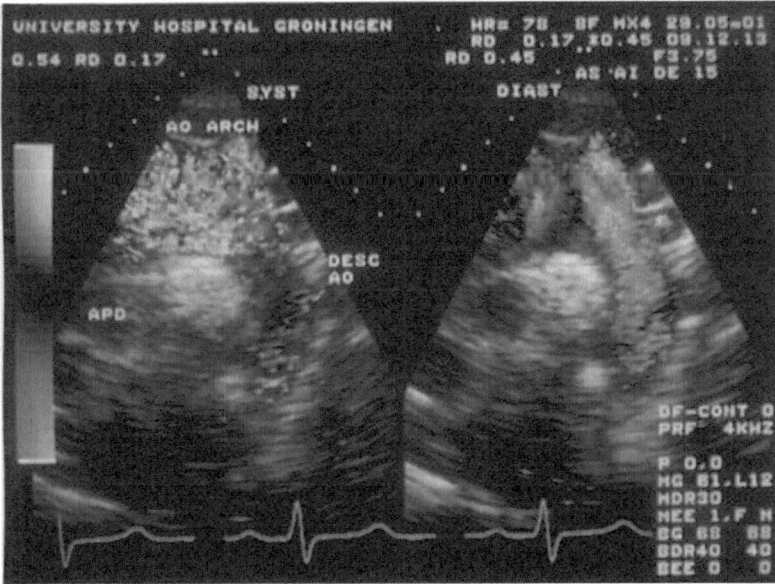

Fig. 8-90. Color Doppler suprasternal view of aortic insufficiency. During systole (left) turbulent colors fill up the whole aortic arch (AO ARCH). During diastole (right) the arch should be black but is red, indicating a backflow from the descending aorta (DESC AO). APD = right pulmonary artery.

Rather good correlations have been found between the area of color Doppler from the apical view in aortic insufficiency and the severity, established with angiography. It should be realized however, that many factors influence the presence, intensity and shape of a color area. Also, the area of contrast on the angiocardiogram depends on several factors (Chapter 6).

From the suprasternal view, reversed flow can be found in the thoracic aorta during diastole, indicating insufficiency (Fig. 8-90). The same feature can be seen in recordings from the femoral artery.

Good colors from aortic insufficiency can often be obtained with TEE (Fig. 8-91).

Indirect features
Aortic ring and root. An obviously normal aortic valve does not exclude aortic insufficiency. The combination can be found in dilatation of the ascending aorta with or without dissection. In long-standing dilatation, the aortic ring also dilates and coaptation of the cusps during diastole is lost, causing insufficiency.

The Marfan syndrome is a generalized abnormality of connective tissue with weakness of the supporting tissues. The patients are characteristically tall with

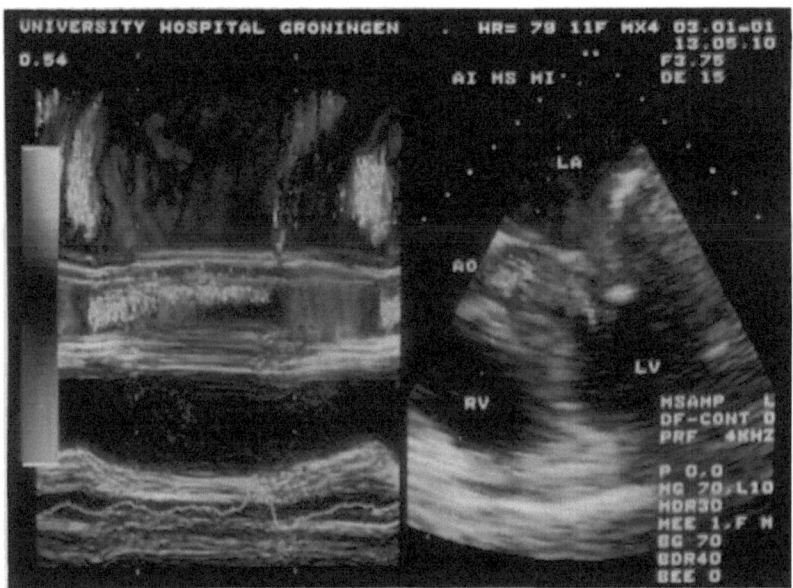

Fig. 8-91. Aortic insufficiency with TEE. In the diastolic frame the LV outflow tract is filled up with turbulent and red colors originating from the aortic valve and proving aortic insufficiency. There is also some degree of mitral stenosis. The M-mode recording shows besides the aortic insufficiency also mitral insufficiency (systolic turbulent colors in the LA).

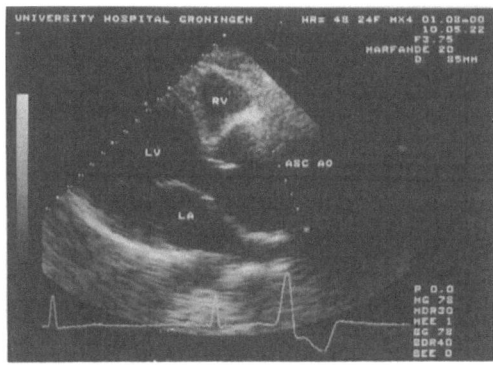

Fig. 8-92. Long axis view of Marfan syndrome. The LV is greatly enlarged. The LA is compressed by an also greatly enlarged aortic root. This enlargement is a well-known cause of aortic insufficiency.

long, thin arms and legs and often have subluxation of the eye lenses. Aortic aneurysm and dissection are possible; especially the aortic root and ascending aorta are dilated (Fig. 8-92). Dilatation can be severe and rupture of the aortic wall is possible. Dilatation of the aortic ring can also be found. The combination causes aortic insufficiency in the presence of a normal-looking valve.

Dissection of the ascending aorta can be found in the long axis view as the ultrasound hits the intima layer perpendicularly. Dissections are futher discussed in Chapter 8, 'thoracic aorta'.

Mitral valve. In aortic insufficiency, a diastolic high-frequency flutter can be found on the AML (Fig. 8-88). This flutter may be 'audible' at the apex of the heart as a diastolic rumble, resembling mitral stenosis (Austin-Flint murmur)

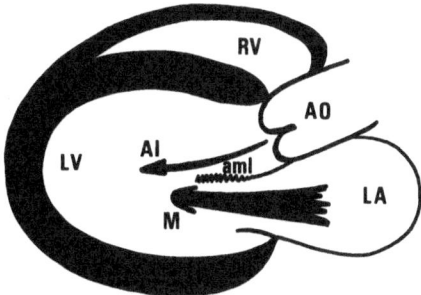

Fig. 8-93. Diagram illustrating the cause of a flutter on the AML in aortic insufficiency. There is a high velocity insufficiency (AI) and a low velocity mitral inflow (M). Between two different velocities a flexible structure will always flutter.

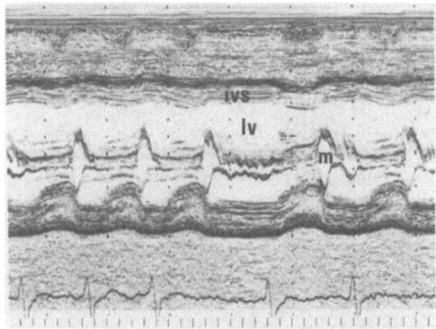

Fig. 8-94. Left parasternal M-mode recording in aortic insufficiency. The mitral valve (m) shows a flutter as well as compression, both caused by aortic insufficiency.

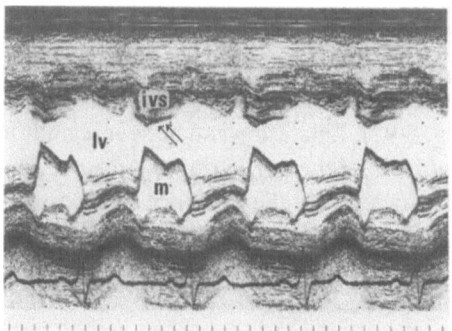

Fig. 8-95. Left parasternal M-mode recording of aortic insufficiency. The LV is slightly enlarged with a good motion pattern. The mitral leaflets (m) are normal without a flutter. Obviously, the direction of the aortic insufficiency is towards the IVS as a flutter is recorded there (arrows).

The flutter is caused by the high flow velocity of the insufficiency that strikes along the ventricular side of the AML, simultaneously with the low flow velocity from ventricular inflow along the atrial side. A smooth AML between two different flow velocities will show a flutter then (Fig. 8-93, 8-94).

This flutter can only be found if the insufficiency flow is directed towards the AML. If the flow is directed towards the IVS, there is no flutter on the AML; in this condition, sometimes a flutter can be recorded from the IVS (Fig. 8-95). This direction-dependent flutter explains the poor correlation between the presence of a flutter and the severity of aortic insufficiency.

Helpful in establishing the severity of aortic insufficiency is the moment of closure of the mitral valve. Normally, the closure is caused by LV contraction and can be recorded on M-mode at the R of the ECG. In severe aortic

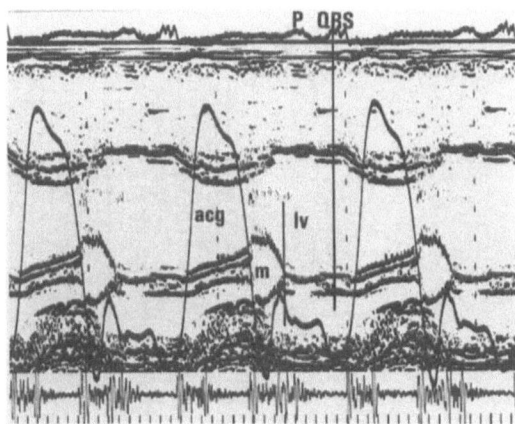

Fig. 8-96. Left parasternal M-mode recording of the mitral valve in aortic insufficiency together with the apexcardiogram (acg). The mitral valve (m) is already closed before the R of ECG, even before the P-wave (P). The closure of the mitral valve coincides with a diastolic sound. From the acg it can be seen that filling of the LV is also impaired after this moment. The LA contracts against a closed valve. The recording indicates very severe aortic insufficiency.

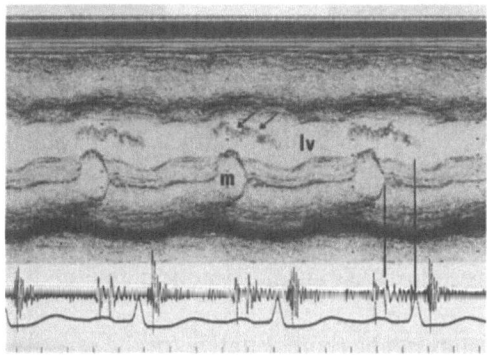

Fig. 8-97. Left parasternal M-mode recording of the mitral valve in aortic insufficiency. The mitral valve (m) is closed far before the R of ECG. A mitral closure sound is recorded on the phonocardiogram. Part of the aortic valve is visible in the LV, indicating aortic valve rupture. The aortic insufficiency is very severe.

insufficiency, the valve is put in a pre-closure position by a massive flow directed towards the AML but also by a quick rise of the LV diastolic pressure to more than the LA pressure. This explains the soft first heart sound that is found in significant aortic insufficiency. The mitral valve can even be closed by the high diastolic LV pressure before the QRS complex. This is always a severe condition. Often atrial contraction is then against the closed mitral valve (Fig. 8-96). Occasionally, the early closure can be recorded as a mitral closure sound before ventricular contraction (Fig. 8-97).

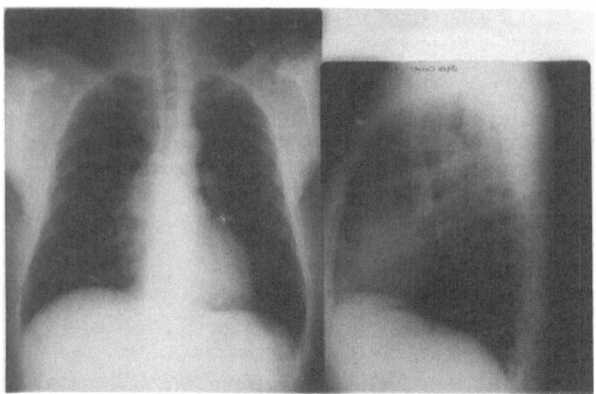

Fig. 8-98. Chest X-ray of a patient with severe aortic insufficiency. If the cardiothoracic ratio (CTR) should be used to evaluate LV enlargement, one could be reassured by this chest X ray: the CTR is 15/32 (< 0.5) but the LV diameters are 72 and 50 mm!

Left ventricle. In significant aortic insufficiency, the LV reacts with dilatation and hypertrophy. Hypertrophy is less important: the finding of a normal LV wall thickness does not exclude severe aortic insufficiency, especially if short standing as in valve rupture caused by endocarditis. Dilatation is diagnosed from the end-diastolic diameter but especially, measurement of the end-systolic LV diameter is important. If end-systolic diameters increase with follow-up examinations, the condition is often severe enough to consider surgery. Several institutions use an end-systolic diameter of 50 mm as a critical value for surgery.

The chest X-ray may not be representative for the severity of LV dilatation. This means that if a cardiothoracic ratio of < 0.5 is found on the chest X-ray (which is considered to be normal) in the presence of aortic insufficiency, a severe dilatation of the LV still may be present (Fig. 8-98).

With a good quality myocardium, the difference between systolic and diastolic diameters is greater than normal as there is volume overload of the ventricle. A normal or subnormal difference in the presence of aortic insufficiency is suggestive for myocardial failure. In ventricular failure the LVEDP increases, which is detected by an enlarged a/H ratio from the ACG (Fig. 8-74).

To be investigated in aortic insufficiency
echocardiography:
– shape of the leaflets, intensity of the echoes from the valve, diastolic flutter;

vegetations, valve rupture (short axis aortic, long axis, TEE)
- LV dimensions (long axis view)
- LV wall thickness (long axis view)

Doppler:
(-slope of the CW signal, $t^1/_2p$ value (apical view))

color Doppler:
(-largest color area (all possible views))

pulse recording:
- a/H ratio (ACG)

MITRAL VALVE

The normal mitral valve

Possible recordings of anatomical normal mitral leaflets

Possible M-mode recordings of anatomical normal mitral leaflets (except for mitral valve prolapse and chordal rupture) with explanations are presented in (Fig. 8-99).

In normal conditions
From both leaflets, the AML is the longest one with the largest leaflet area. The area of attachment to the mitral ring, however, is smaller than for the PML (Fig. 8-100).

The AML is recorded better than the PML. Often it is the first moving structure on the echocardiogram which is helpful in image orientation. From the long axis view, the opened AML is hit perpendicularly, providing good echoes. The PML is shorter. During ventricular diastole, the valve is near to the LVPW. During ventricular systole, the valve is almost in line with the ultrasound beams and thus less good visible than the AML.

During diastole, both leaflets move in opposite directions (Fig. 8-101).

The valve opens at D. The initial opening is fast and the widest leaflet separation is at E. Then the valve tends to close, initially fast and after F less quickly. If the duration of diastole is long enough, separation again augments. After that, the valve is opened again by atrial contraction (A). The amplitude of the A-wave is less than from the initial opening at point E. In higher heart rates, only the E and A waves are visible. If heart rates are still higher, just a single opening wave is found from the mitral valve. The valve is closed at point C by LV contraction. In the long axis view, the closure line of the leaflets (C-D) is a straight line that moves towards the transducer during systole.

The Doppler evaluation of the normal mitral valve in normal conditions is discussed in Chapter 7.

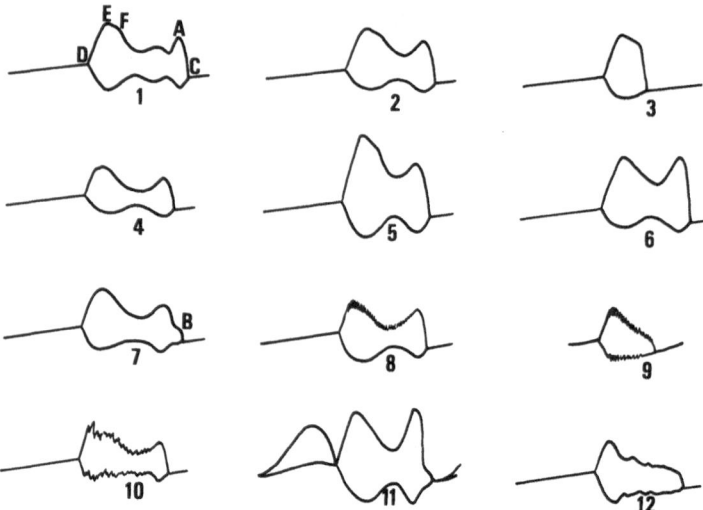

Fig. 8-99. Possible recordings of anatomical normal mitral leaflets, except for mitral valve prolapse and for all aspects of chordal rupture. In all examples except for 12, normal sinus rhythm with normal PQ time is assumed.

1. normal aspect. The valve opens at D when the rapid filling period of the LV starts. This is a passive filling by LV relaxation. The highest amplitude in this phase is at E. The E-F slope represents the early diastolic closing velocity. Increased LV stiffness may decrease the E-F slope, as does mitral stenosis. The F-A period is the slow filling phase of the LV. Point A reflects atrial contraction. The valve closes at C by LV contraction.
2. normal at a higher heart rate than 1
3. normal aspect at a higher heart rate than 2
4. smaller amplitude: hypovolemia
5. wide separation: hypervolemia
6. large A wave: impaired LV diastolic function
7. delayed closure point B: increased LVEDP
8. diastolic flutter AML: aortic insufficiency. This regular high frequency flutter has to be differentiated from the irregular low frequency flutter as found in chordal rupture and as seen in 10
9. diastolic flutter AML with compression and early closure without effect of atrial contraction: severe aortic insufficiency
10. coarse flutter on both leaflets: obstruction by a LA tumor or cor triatriatum, chordal rupture
11. with SAM, large A wave and B point: HOCM
12. no A wave as in atrial fibrillation

In abnormal conditions

Besides heart rate and heart rhythm, the diastolic aspect of the normal mitral valve depends on several factors.

If a small volume of blood passes the valve with a low velocity, it opens less wide than normal.

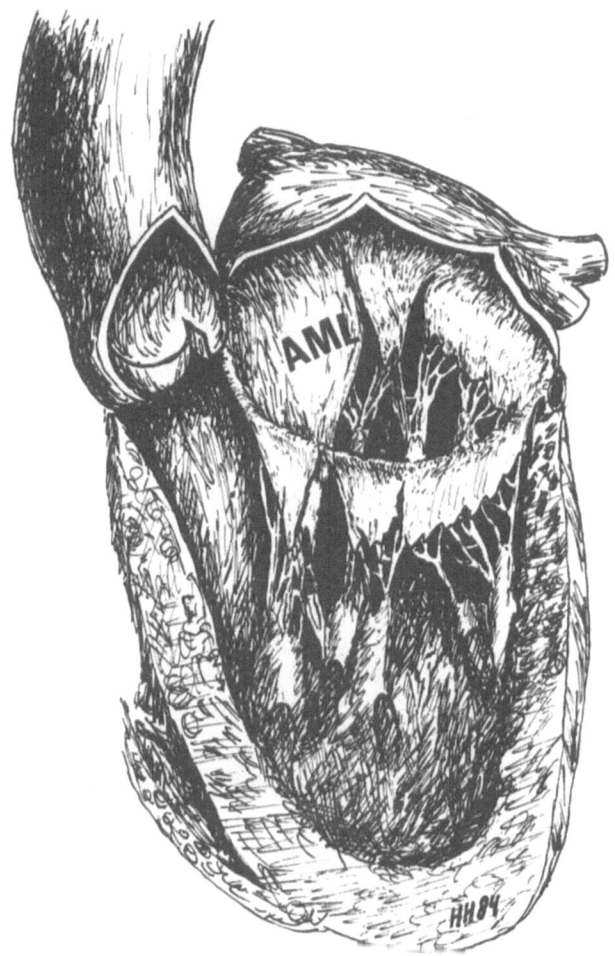

Fig. 8-100. Illustration of the mitral valve, LV and aorta. The AML is the largest leaflet. The PML, usually consists of three parts. The PML has a larger area of attachment to the valve ring than the AML.

If a large volume of blood passes the valve with a high velocity, as in large stroke volumes and in significant mitral insufficiency, the valve opens wider than normal. In this condition, a 'physiological' diastolic flutter can be record-ed, usually from the PML (Fig. 8-102) which has to be differentiated from the flutter caused by chordal rupture.

In impaired diastolic function of the LV, the initial blood flow velocity through the mitral ostium is low and leaflet separation is smaller than normal. The amplitude of A may be larger than from E.

In increased LVEDP, closure of the mitral valve may be delayed. This is

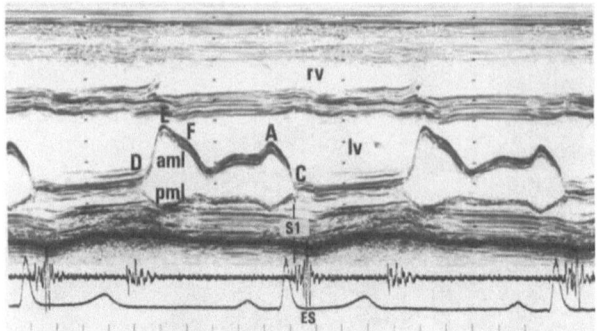

Fig. 8-101. Normal mitral valve. See text for explanation. C coincides with a soft mitral closure sound (S1, vertical line), and is immediately followed by an ejection sound of the aorta (ES).

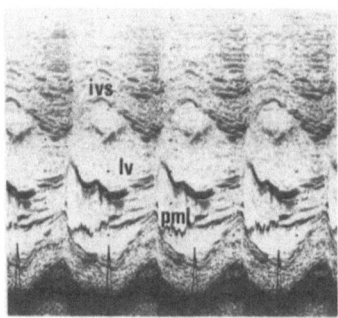

Fig. 8-102. Parasternal M-mode recording of the mitral valve of a 15 year old boy. A coarse flutter is recorded from the PML without any abnormality of the heart and valves. As there was no murmur, the condition was easily differentiated from chordal rupture.

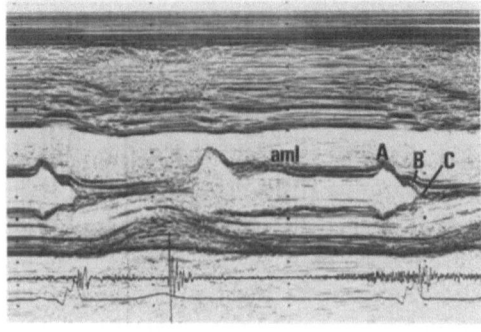

Fig. 8-103. Parasternal M-mode recording of the mitral valve in HCM at a paper speed of 100 mm/sec. B is caused by increased LVEDP.

recorded as prolongation of the A-C interval in the presence of a normal P-Q interval. The closure line between A and C is interrupted at point B (Fig. 8-103).

In aortic insufficiency, the AML may be compressed with a diastolic flutter on the AML and/or an early closure. This is further discussed in the section aortic insufficiency.

In intra-atrial obstruction caused by tumors, the impaired flow through the mitral ostium causes decreased valve separation. In cor triatriatum, an obstructing membrane in the LA causes a jet towards the mitral valve, visible as flutters on both leaflets.

In LV outflow tract obstruction by HOCM, the systolic motion pattern of the mitral valve may be distorted by a systolic anterior motion of the AML and/or chordae. Mitral insufficiency is then possible, in the presence of a normal mitral valve. This is further discussed in the section left ventricle.

The regular wave pattern of an atrial flutter is often reflected on the mitral valve recording (Fig. 8-104). Irregular wave patterns (sometimes resembling much those from atrial flutter) can be found in atrial fibrillation (Fig. 8-105).

The abnormal mitral valve

Mitral insufficiency

Mitral insufficiency is a volume overload for the LV and the LA. Depending on the severity, LV hypertrophy and dilatation may develop. The LA volume

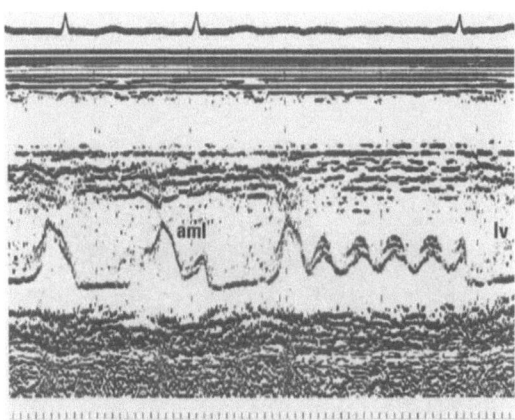

Fig. 8-104. M-mode recording of the AML in atrial flutter. The atrial contractions are reflected in the AML.

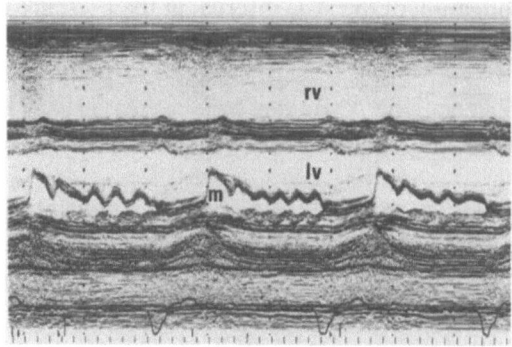

Fig. 8-105. M-mode recording of the mitral valve in atrial fibrillation. The diastolic wave pattern of the leaflets largely resembles that from atrial fibrillation, but is not regular.

overload causes LA dilatation. Both overloads may cause atrial and ventricular rhythm disturbances. In LV failure, LVEDP also increases resulting in pressure and volume overload of the LA. Blood pressure and blood volume in the lungs also increase. Thus, the most important complaints of the patient are dyspnea and fatigue on physical exertion or even at rest. The pulmonary artery pressure rises and pulmonary hypertension may develop. This may be followed by tricuspid regurgitation.

Diagnosis and severity
With echocardiography, the LV may be diffusely thickened with an exaggerated, enthousiastic motion pattern. LA and LV both enlarge. Mitral insufficiency can be detected with CW from the apical view (Fig. 8-106).

If detection is difficult, mitral insufficiency may be less severe than if detected easily. Some institutions use the area of color flow as a criterion for the degree of mitral insufficiency (Fig. 8-107). The intensity, shape and depth

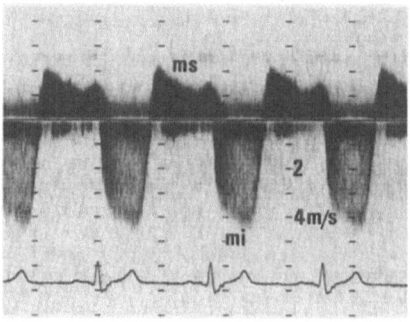

Fig. 8-106. Apical CW recording of combined mitral insufficiency (mi) and mitral stenosis (ms).

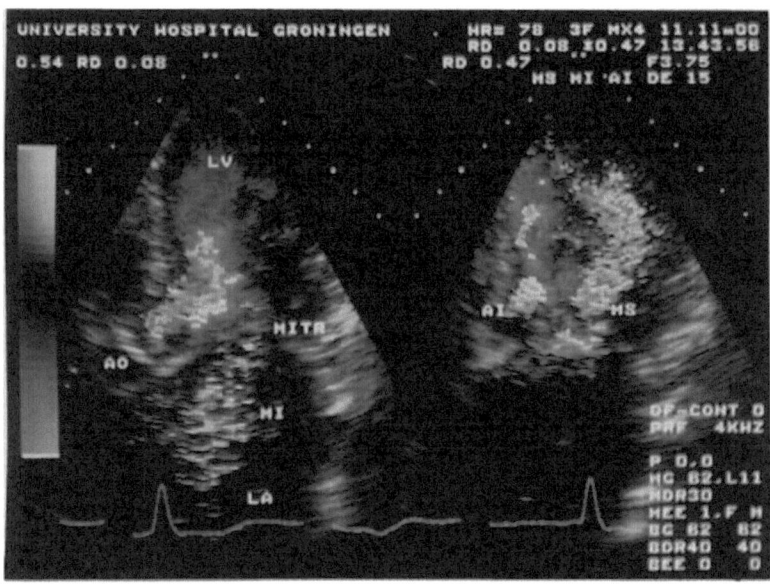

Fig. 8-107. Apical color Doppler recording of mitral insufficiency (MI), mitral stenosis (MS) and aortic insufficiency (AI). The area of the colors in the LA are sometimes used to express the severity of mitral insufficiency. Note the angle between the direction of mitral inflow and the position of the transducer. MITR = mitral valve, AO = aortic valve.

of a color flow jet, however, depend on many factors (Chapter 6).

With color, many minor insufficiencies are missed or cannot be found: the valve is far away from the transducer and the mitral valve itself can also interfere with the intensity of the colors in the LA. Often a blue color can be found in the LV during systole, that 'stops' abruptly against the mitral valve without colors in the LA. This is an indirect proof of mitral insufficiency that could not be visualized with color in the LA because of interference of the valve itself.

With TEE and color Doppler, high quality pictures are obtained from mitral insufficiency, often together with their causes (Fig. 8-108).

Causes
Mitral insufficiency may be congenital. In ASD I a cleft AML can be found. Other causes of mitral insufficiency with an abnormal mitral valve are mitral valve prolapse, chordal rupture, inflammation (rheumatic, endocarditis) and occasionally, tumors.

Mitral valve prolapse (MVP). The typical auscultation of an MVP is an early, mid- or late-systolic click at the apex, followed by a late-systolic murmur.

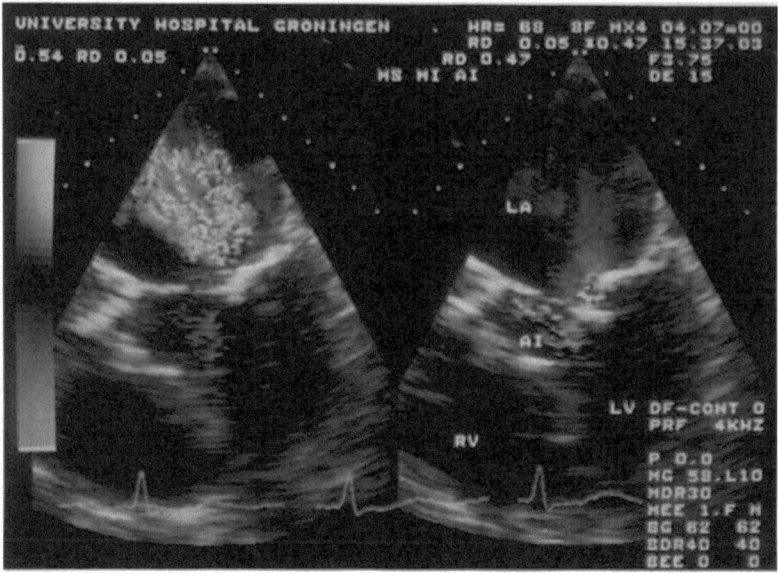

Fig. 8-108. TEE recording of mitral stenosis and insufficiency and aortic insufficiency (AI). During systole (left) bright turbulent colors, caused by mitral insufficiency, fill a large part of the LA. During diastole the blue color in the LA indicates flow towards the LV; the red color in the LV outflow tract proves aortic insufficiency.

However, with echocardiography, an MVP can be found without these auscultatory signs. On the other hand, auscultation can prove an MVP that cannot be found with echocardiography.

A patient with MVP may have complaints such as palpitations, chest pain, dyspnea, fatigue, dizziness and syncope. Sudden death has occassionally been described. Also, the patient may have no complaints, or may have the same complaints as in mitral insufficiency due to other causes.

MVP is more often found in women. Depending on the criteria, MVP can be found in about 4% of the normal population.

In MVP, part of the AML and/or PML prolapses into the LA during the whole or a part of ventricular systole (Fig. 8-109).

MVP may be caused by very large valve leaflets, (relatively) too long chordae, a small mitral ring, an abnormal shape of the annulus, an abnormal change in shape of the annulus during systole, an abnormal contraction pattern of a papillary muscle and/or the LV wall, abnormal dimensions of the LV or by a combination of factors. The presence or absence of an MVP also depends on the heart rate (size of the LV!), position of the patient and the use of drugs such as β-blocking agents. An MVP may disappear by the use of β-blocking agents as they lower the heart rate and thus enlarge the LV. The presence of mitral

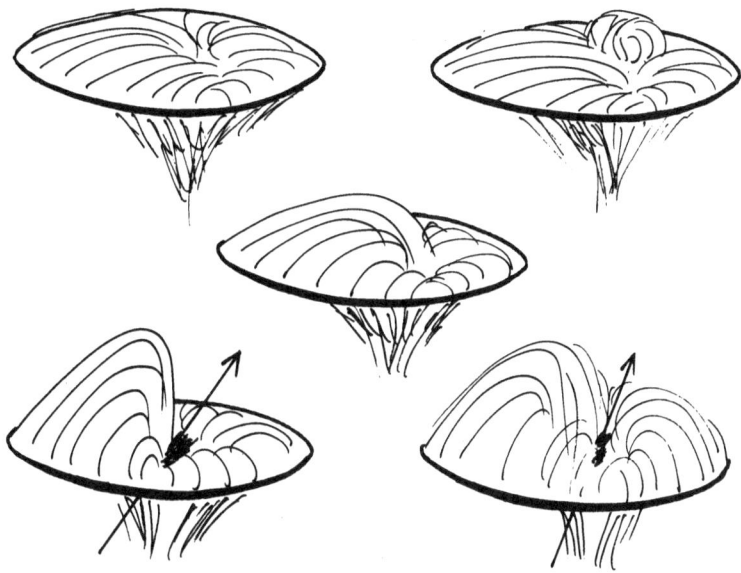

Fig. 8-109. Schematic representation of a normal mitral valve and of various types of MVP. The normal mitral valve has a large AML (left) and a smaller PML (upper left). An MVP can be localized to e.g. a posterior part of the PML (upper right). In the middle a prolapse of the AML is seen. If the prolapse of the AML is deeper (lower left), mitral insufficiency may be present. The lower right picture shows prolapse of both leaflets with insufficiency.

insufficiency in MVP also depends on these factors. Usually, insufficiency is not severe if MVP is late-systolic.

As the presence of a specific apical murmur is often the reason for echocardiography, the dependency of a prolapse murmur on LV volume is illustrated in Fig. 8-110.

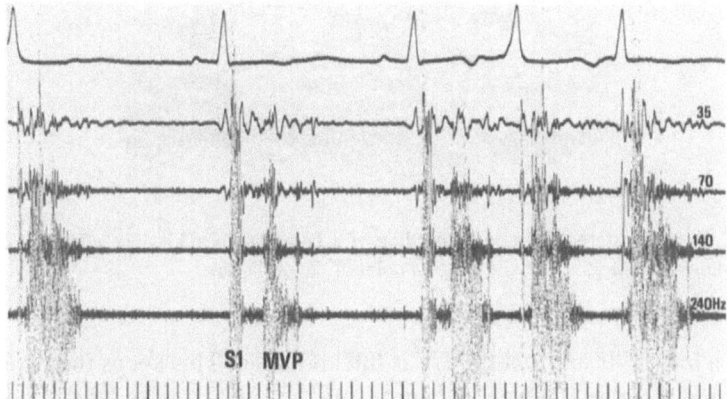

Fig. 8-110. Phonocardiogram at the apex of an MVP. The cut-off frequencies are 35, 70, 140 and 240 Hz. S1 = mitral closure sound. See text for explanation.

156

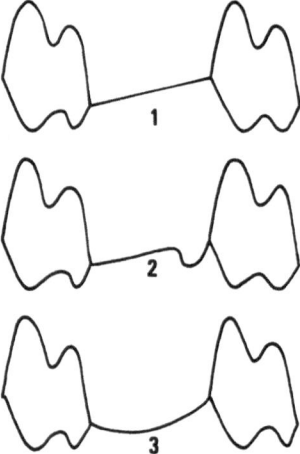

Fig. 8-111. Schematic possibilities of MVP on the M-mode recording. The normal systolic closure line of the mitral leaflets is a straight line with an anterior motion during systole; this pattern does not exclude an MVP (1). A late-systolic downward motion is typical for a late-systolic prolapse (2). A holosystolic prolapse is illustrated in 3.

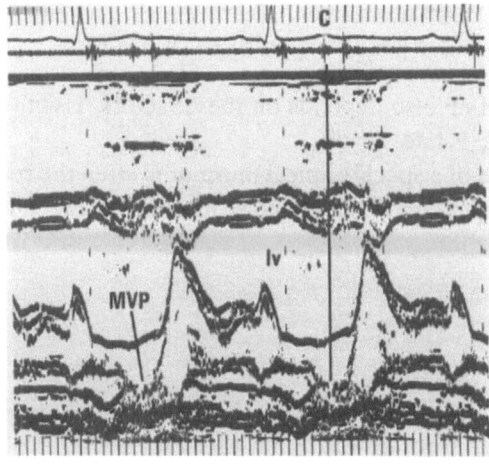

Fig. 8-112. Left parasternal M-mode recording of a late-systolic MVP. The click (C) on the phonocardiogram coincides with the deepest point of the prolapse.

After a long R-R interval the LV is full and large. This keeps the papillary muscles and chordae at a great distance from the mitral ring and there is only a slight possibilty of mitral valve prolapse: only a late-systolic murmur is recorded. After a few short R-R intervals the LV is much smaller and the papillary

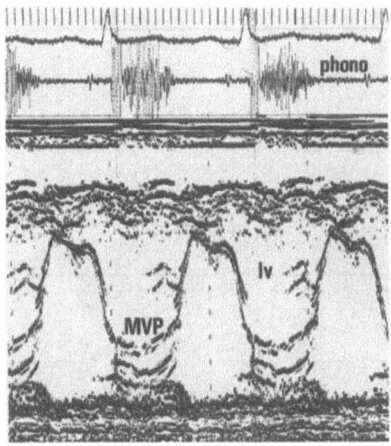

Fig. 8-113. Left parasternal M-mode recording of a holosystolic prolapse. A holosystolic murmur is recorded on the phonocardiogram (phono), proving mitral insufficiency.

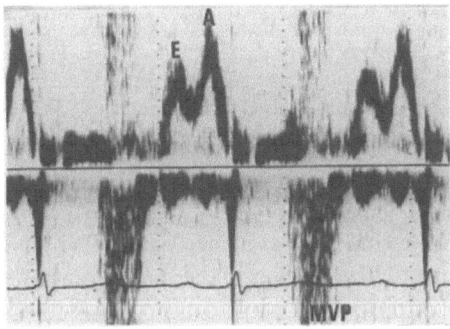

Fig. 8-114. Apical PD of an MVP. A late-systolic negative Doppler signal indicates mitral insufficiency caused by MVP. In this patient A is taller than E, indicating impaired LV diastolic function.

muscles and chordae are closer to the mitral ring: the prolapse starts earlier in systole and is on the right of the recording even holosystolic.

All these factors explain how it is possible that an MVP may have been heard in the outpatients clinic can fail to be diagnosed with echocardiography. More often, however, MVP is diagnosed with echocardiography, without the auscultatory features of a systolic click and/or murmur.

On the M-mode recording, the closure line shows a holosystolic or late-systolic downward motion from the parasternal view. Several types of M-mode recordings can be found (Fig. 8-111, 8-112, 8-113). Pulsed Doppler is an excellent tool for the detection of mitral insufficiency caused by MVP (Fig. 8-114).

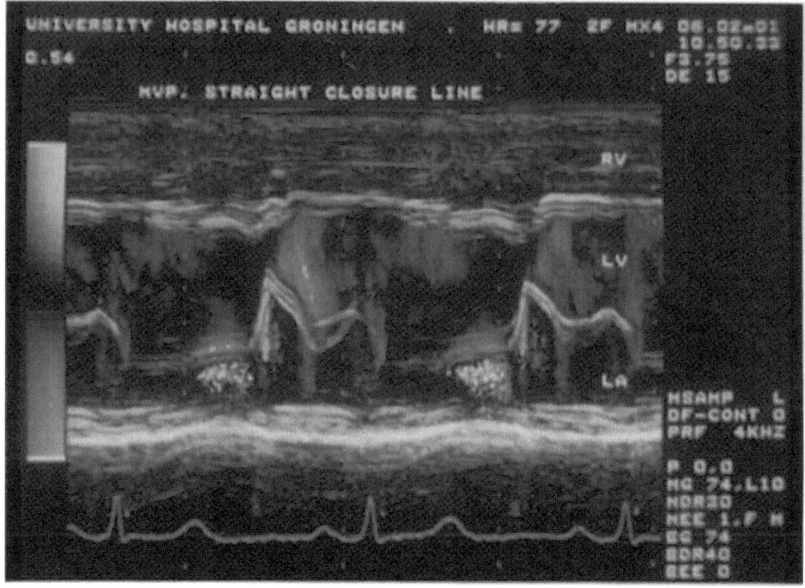

Fig. 8-115. Left parasternal M-mode recording of the mitral valve. There is a straight closure line: an MVP is not found with echocardiography. However, at the same time an end-systolic yellow-green color proves mitral insufficiency, caused by prolapse.

The absence of a holo- or late-systolic downward motion from the parasternal view does not exclude the presence of MVP (Fig. 8-115): only a small part of the valve, outside the section plane may prolapse.

Criteria for MVP differ between institutions. There is a spectrum between apparently normal valves and MVP. Usually, a downward motion of more than 3 mm is used as a criterion. Additional to the parasternal view, the apical view may be useful. Several MVP's have been found from this view that could not been diagnosed from the parasternal view.

Also, with TEE an MVP which is not detectable from other views, is sometimes found.

Chordal rupture (CR). CR develops spontaneously or is caused by endocarditis, rheumatic heart disease, hypertension, chest trauma, physical exertion and mitral valve prolapse. The resulting mitral insufficiency is often significant, but may be minor, and CR can exist for many years without necessary intervention. It can also be acute, severe and life-threatening. The symptoms are the same as for mitral insufficiency without CR.

Patients may have no complaints or may have symptoms such as fatigue, dyspnea and rhythm disturbances.

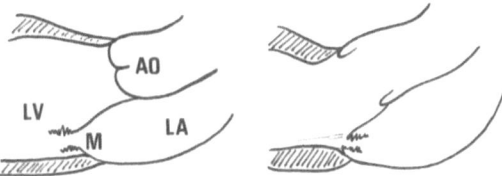

Fig. 8-116. Echocardiographic criteria for chordal rupture if a mitral insufficiency murmur is present. See text for explanation. AO = aorta, M = mitral valve.

An apical thrill is found in the majority of patients. The thrill is often palpable during the echo-examination with the transducer at the apex. If so the examiner should think of the posssibility of CR. It is important to find or exclude CR as a cause of severe mitral insufficiency, as the surgeon can be informed in advance and repair -if possible- the valve instead of replacing it.

Criteria for CR (Fig. 8-116) – if there is mitral insufficiency – are
- a systolic flutter of the mitral valve
- a diastolic, inconstant, low frequency flutter similar to the pattern made by an irregular saw blade. This flutter has to be differentiated from the low frequency flutter that can be seen in case of atrial fibrillation which does not have a sharply pointed aspect. It also excludes a flutter caused by aortic regurgitation which has a high frequency and is often regular.

Examples of M-mode echocardiographic recordings of CR from the parasternal long axis view are presented in Fig. 8-117, 8-118, 8-119.

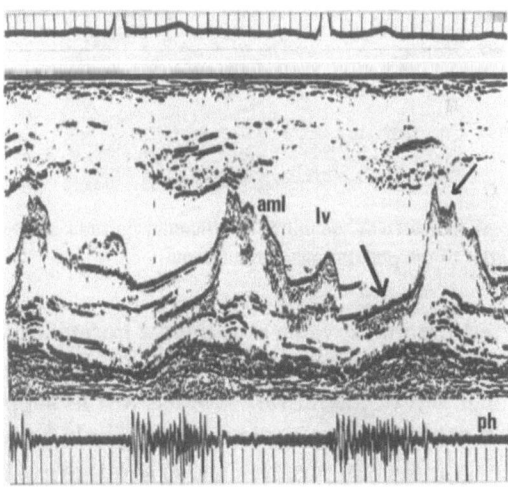

Fig. 8-117. CR of the aml and pml, indicated by the mitral insufficiency murmur on the phonocardiogram (ph) and coarse, irregular flutters on both mitral leaflets (arrows).

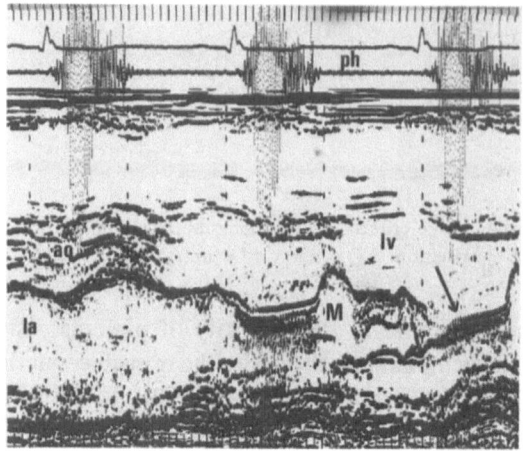

Fig. 8-118. CR of the mitral valve (M), indicated by the mitral insufficiency murmur on the phonocardiogram (ph) and a flutter on the closure line of the valve (arrow). ao = aorta.

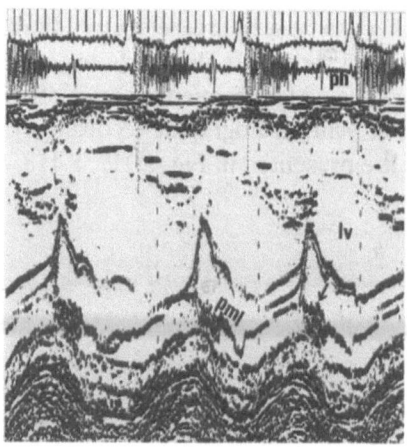

Fig. 8-119. CR of the pml, indicated by the mitral insufficiency murmur on the phonocardiogram (ph) and the coarse flutter of the pml during systole (arrow).

Besides the flutter, the mitral valve may have a normal aspect but vegetations can be found in the presence of endocarditis (Fig. 8-120).

If only a very small part of the mitral valve has lost its support, a flutter is difficult to find. All possible transducer positions should be used to find the flutter. TEE provides far the best position: a very good view of the mitral valve is obtained and this technique is very helpful in the diagnosis of CR (Fig. 8-121). Also, with TEE the type and technique of valve repair can often be predicted.

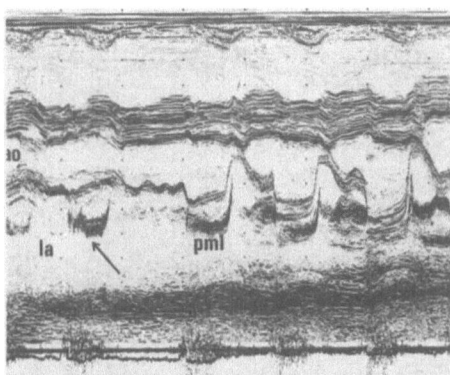

Fig. 8-120. Parasternal long axis M-mode sweep from the aortic valve (ao) to the LV. In the LA already, a fluttering echogenic mass indicates the presence of CR of the pml with vegetations (arrow).

CW Doppler is helpful in the diagnosis of mitral insufficiency. With color, the location of CR is easier to find. The direction of flow may vary, depending on the location of CR. Often, CR of the PML shows a flow directed along the atrial side of the AML and along the aortic root (Fig. 8-122).

The severity of mitral insufficiency caused by CR should be estimated and measured as generally done in mitral insufficiency. It should be noted however, that in short standing severe CR, the LA still has a normal diameter and forceful contractions are found from a normal sized LV.

Endocarditis. From the cardiac valves, the mitral valve is most often involved in endocarditis. One reason is that the pressure differences across valves is the greatest between LV and LA which may more readily cause damage of the

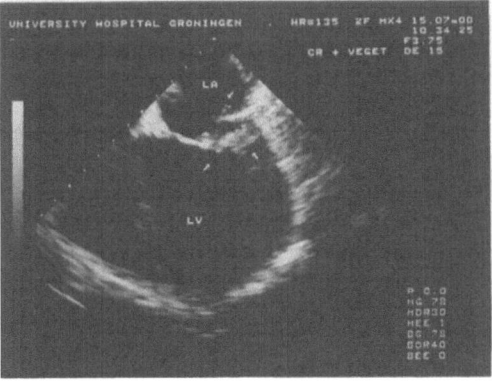

Fig. 8-121. TEE of CR. CR of the pml is visible in the LA (arrow in LA). Large vegetations are found at the aml (arrows in LV).

162

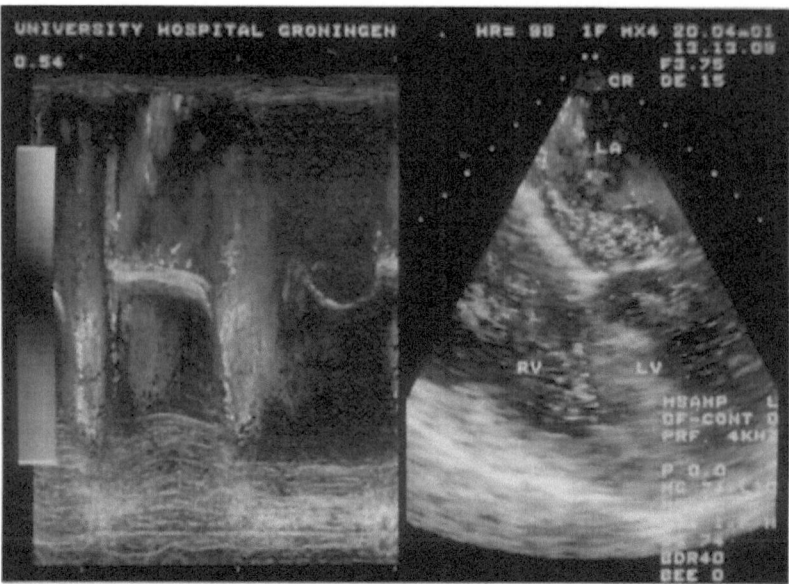

Fig. 8-122. TEE sector and M-mode recording of CR of the pml. The turbulent and red colors in the LA indicate a flow direction along the atrial side of the aml and along the inter-atrial septum, as is often found in CR of the pml. On the M-mode recording a systolic flutter is visible, caused by CR.

leaflets. Another reason may be that 'physiologic' insufficiency is often seen from the normal mitral valve and hardly or not at all from the normal aortic valve. Mitral valve prolapse is a well known cause of endocarditis (Fig. 8-123).

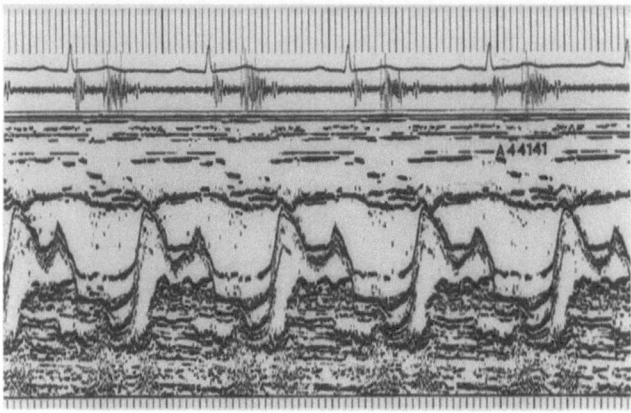

Fig. 8-123. Late-systolic mitral valve prolapse, recorded on M-mode as a deep end-systolic downward motion of the mitral closure line; it is also visible from the phonocardiogram as a late-systolic murmur. The pml is thickened, caused by vegetations.

Echocardiographically, endocarditis can be suspected if vegetation-like structures can be recorded at the valve. Mitral insufficiency is almost always present. It should be kept in mind that very small vegetations are not detected with echocardiography. Consequently, endocarditis cannot be excluded when vegetations are not found.

Valve rupture (Fig. 8-124, 8-125) and/or chordal rupture can be found, caused by weakening of the structures.

The ideal position for examining vegetations and mitral insufficiency is with TEE, with which a good quality recording of the mitral valve is obtained. (Fig. 8-125, 8-126).

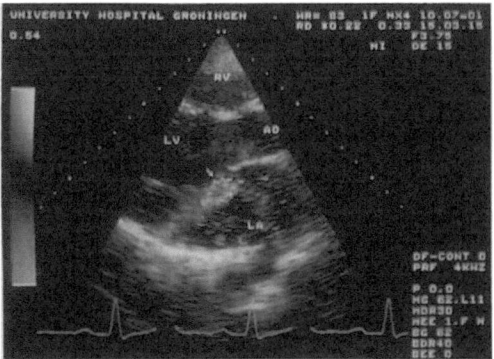

Fig. 8-124. Systolic frame of a parasternal long axis view. The blue area with aliasing (arrow) indicates mitral insufficiency. The origin of the insufficiency however is not at the level of the mitral closure line, but above this area. This makes perforation of the aml highly possible.

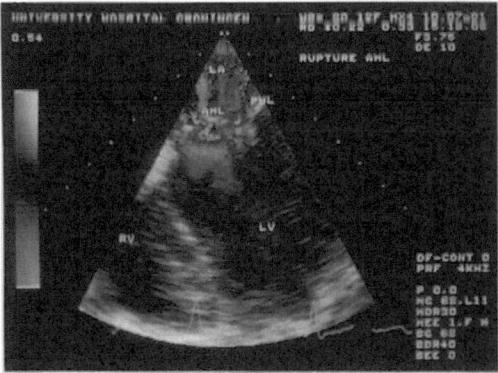

Fig. 8-125. TEE of the same patient as Fig. 8-124. Mitral insufficiency is visible at two levels: a broad dark red area with aliasing in the LV just below the aml with turbulent colors right through the aml and in the LA prove a valve rupture. Another but small dark red area in the LV at the closure line of the leaflets indicates minor insufficiency there.

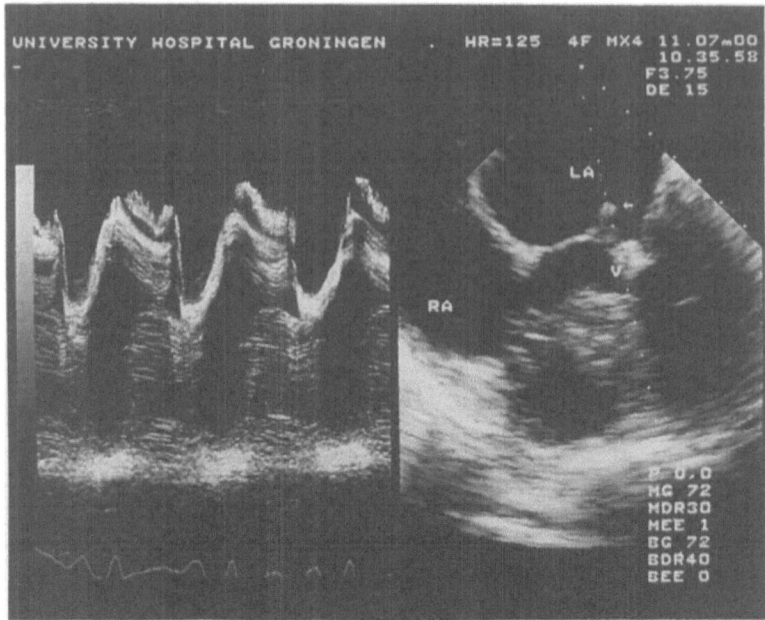

Fig. 126. TEE of mitral valve vegetations. Vegetations are recorded from the aml (arrow) and from the pml (V).

To be investigated in mitral insufficiency
echocardiography:
- LV dimensions (long axis view)
- LV wall thickness (long axis view)
- M-mode from the mitral valve: late closure (increased LVEDP)
- aspect of the mitral valve: normal, thickened, MVP, CR, vegetations?
- LA dimensions (long axis and apical view)
Doppler:
- presence of mitral insufficiency (apical view)
- flow velocities, E/A ratio (apical view)
color Doppler:
- area of color? Depth of color flow jet? (apical view)
- (+CW) RV peak pressure (short axis aortic, apical view)
- IVC diameters during respiration
TEE:
- aspect of the mitral valve
- color flow direction; color area
pulse recording:
- a/H ratio (ACG)

Mitral stenosis

The main cause of mitral stenosis is rheumatic heart disease. Occasionally, mitral stenosis is congenital. The mitral valve can also be obstructed by a LA tumor. The narrowed ostium causes an LA overload, with a dimished LV stroke volume.

The physical findings and the complaints depend on the severity of the obstruction. The apex impulse is small, occasionally with a diastolic thrill. At auscultation, a mitral opening snap can be heard, followed by a diastolic rumble.In severe mitral stenosis, the IIP sound may be loud, indicating pulmonary hypertension. Tricuspid insufficiency may be present, caused by dilatation of the RV and the tricuspid ring.

At rest, the patient may have no complaints. During physical exertion, the filling time for the LV can be too short and the stroke volume of the LV consequently too small. Dyspnea and fatigue may develop. As in the enlarged LA the blood flow velocities are low, thrombus formation -also in sinus rhythm- is possible if the patient is not treated with anti-coagulants. Embolization is possible from these thrombi. The patient may have serious symptoms caused by embolization towards the brain or towards other peripheral arteries.

Usually, atrial fibrillation is found in mitral stenosis. Sinus rhythm, however, can be maintained for many years. Often, the change from sinus rhythm to atrial fibrillation is the moment that the patient complains for the first time since heart rate in untreated atrial fibrillation is often higher than in sinus rhythm.

It has become increasingly important to visualize the stenotic mitral valve as well as possible since it may have therapeutic consequences. In severe mitral stenosis, the decision can be made depending on the aspect of the mitral valve to replace the valve, repair it or to dilate it with a balloon.

Diagnosis and severity
With echocardiography, a stenotic mitral valve is detected easily from the long axis, short axis and apical views. From the long axis view, the normal motion pattern of the AML is changed: the valve shows a straight downslope after initial opening. In severe mitral stenosis, the A-wave is hardly or no longer visible, but usually atrial fibrillation is found in severe mitral stenosis. Characteristic is an anterior motion of the PML during diastole, more or less parallel to the AML. Often, the leaflets are thickened (Fig. 8-127). Leaflet separation is diminished; measurements from leaflet separation, however, may underestimate the significance of mitral stenosis (Fig. 8-128): if the stenotic mitral valve is 'dome-shaped' (see aortic stenosis, Fig. 8-66), leaflet separation is not representative for the ostium area.

The severity of mitral stenosis can be roughly estimated from the size of the

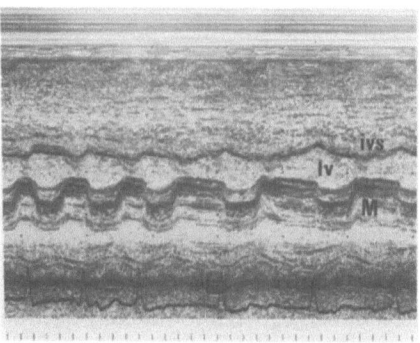

Fig. 8-127. Left parasternal M-mode recording of mitral stenosis. The leaflets of the mitral valve (M) are thickened and the aml and pml cannot be identified separately. There is atrial fibrillation.

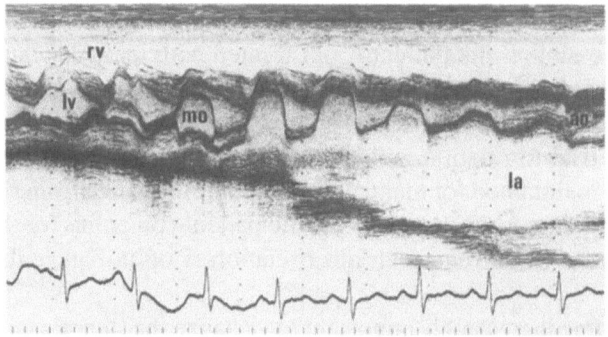

Fig. 8-128. Parasternal long axis sweep from LV to aortic valve (ao). The pml initially moves downwards and leaves a rather large leaflet separation and an acceptable 'mitral ostium' (mo). The severity of mitral stenosis would be under-estimated if this criterion was used. The leaflet separation was caused by a 'dome shaped' mitral valve. Mitral stenosis in this patient appeared to be severe which is also reflected by the very small LV and the enlarged LA.

LA and from the dimensions and the motion pattern of the LV. The LV relaxes slowly in significant mitral stenosis. The LA emptying index can be used as a parameter for impaired LV filling. The LA is enlarged, measured from at least two directions. LA enlargement, however, can also be found with a normal mitral valve (section left atrium).

For the measurement of the severity of mitral stenosis, several methods are used. The mitral ostium area could be calculated from a tracing of the mitral ostium from a frozen sector image (Fig. 8-129). Calcifications of the valve however, nearly always prevent accurate measurement of the ostium area. Routinely, this measurement is barely feasable. It should be realized that such a fixed, anatomical ostium area is not the same as the dynamic, physiologic

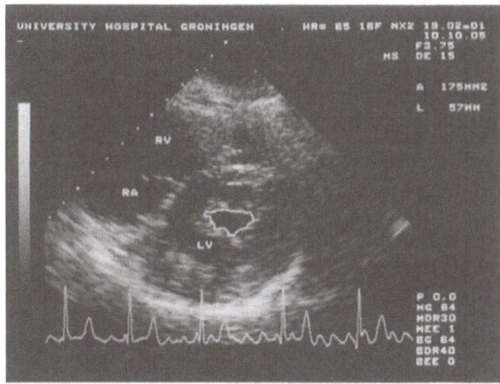

Fig. 8-129. Parasternal short axis view of the LV at the level of the mitral ostium in mitral stenosis. In the absence of calcifications the anatomical ostium area could be measured: 175 mm² in this valve. This is not the same area as measured with cardiac catheterization which is a 'dynamic' area.

ostium area (derived from pressures and cardiac output) that is mostly used as an indication for surgery. Also, the anatomical ostium area is only one parameter for estimating the severity of mitral stenosis: the complaints of the patient and the presence or absence of pulmonary hypertension are important. The main purpose of measurements is to confirm or exclude the possibility that complaints indeed originate from mitral stenosis.

More accurate measurements of the severity of mitral stenosis are possible with Doppler. The best Doppler signal is obtained from the apical view. During diastole, the LV inflow is more or less directed towards the transducer and the Doppler signal is positive. The signal strongly resembles the M-mode pattern of the stenotic mitral valve (Fig. 8-130).

Various measurements can be made from the CW signal: the peak pressure

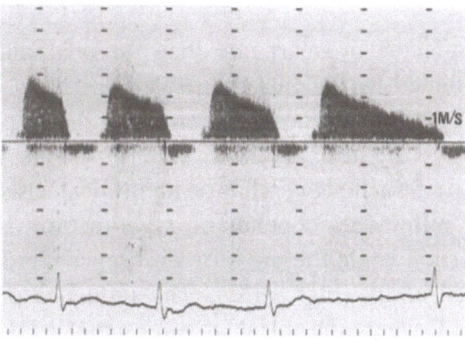

Fig. 8-130. Usual apical CW recording of mitral stenosis. The recording largely resembles the M-mode echocardiogram of a stenotic mitral valve. The peak pressure difference is $4 \times 2.8^2 = 31$ mm Hg, with a heart rate of about 70 b/min.

difference, the pressure halftime ($t^1/_2$p) and the mean pressure difference; The mitral ostium area can be calculated from the $t^1/_2$p. None of them is ideal.

The peak pressure difference is obtained from the highest early diastolic flow velocity with the simplified Bernoulli formula. It is the easiest measurement that can be made from the Doppler signal, but it is affected by cardiac output and heart rate. If mitral regurgitation is also present, peak pressure differences rise and no longer reflect the mitral ostium area. However, the measured obstruction is present.

The $t^1/_2$p is the time required for the peak diastolic pressure to decrease to half its value (Fig. 8-131).

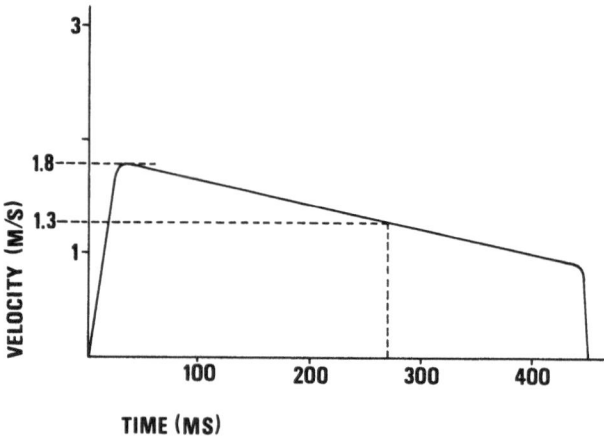

Fig. 8-131. Method of calculation of the $t^1/_2$p value. The peak velocity of the Doppler signal is 1.8 m/sec in the example. The peak pressure difference is $p = 4 \times 1.8^2 = 13$ mm Hg. Thus $^1/_2$p = 6.5 mm Hg. When 6.5 mm Hg = $4v^2$, v = 1.3 m/sec. This velocity is reached after 270 ms, which is the $t^1/_2$p value or $t^1/_2$ time.

The $t^1/_2$p is less affected by heart rate than the peak and mean pressure difference. It is obtained by dividing the peak velocity by $\sqrt{2}$ (peak velocity/1.4). The time between the peak velocity and the $t^1/_2$p velocity is then measured. The $t^1/_2$p for the normal mitral valve is < 60 ms, in mitral stenosis 100-400 ms. The $t^1/_2$p value, however, has no theoretical basis, is influenced by the initial pressure difference, depends on LV function, shows a decrease during physical exertion while the pressure difference increases and can not always be calculated easily (Fig. 8-132). The influence of LV function is illustrated in Fig. 8-133 where the apical Doppler signal in DCM with a normal mitral valve is shown: the signal is almost identical with that from Fig. 8-130 of mitral stenosis. Only the velocities differ.

The mitral ostium area can be derived from the $t^1/_2$p using the empirical

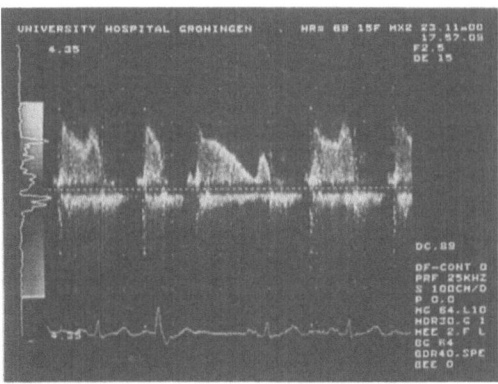

Fig. 8-132. Apical CW recording of the mitral valve in atrial fibrillation. This Figure shows that $t^1/_2p$ values are not always easy to calculate.

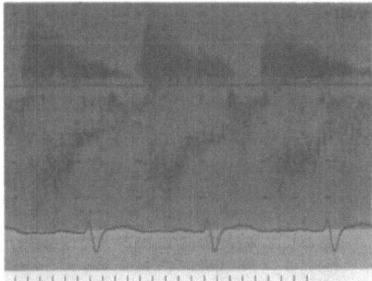

Fig. 8-133. Apical CW Doppler signal from the mitral valve area in DCM. The shape of this signal is suggestive for mitral stenosis; the $t^1/_2p$ value is abnormal and almost the same as from Fig. 8-130. Only the peak pressure differences are not the same: 2.3 mm Hg (heart rate 66 b/min) and 31 mm Hg respectively.

formula MOA $= 220/t^1/_2p$. Thus, for the calculation of the mitral ostium area the same problems are met as mentioned for $t^1/_2p$ measurements; it should be noted that – with this measurement – the ostium area would be larger during physical exertion than at rest! At the same time, the peak pressure difference increases.

The mean pressure difference can be calculated by measuring flow velocities at several points of the curve; the pressure difference is calculated from each point and the mean pressure difference is calculated from these values. The flow velocity curve can also be traced and the machine calculates the mean pressure difference automatically. With this method, however, mean pressure differences can be almost the same in different patients, whereas calculated mitral valve areas differ greatly (Fig. 8-134, 8-135). The mean pressure difference is also influenced by heart rate and mitral insufficiency.

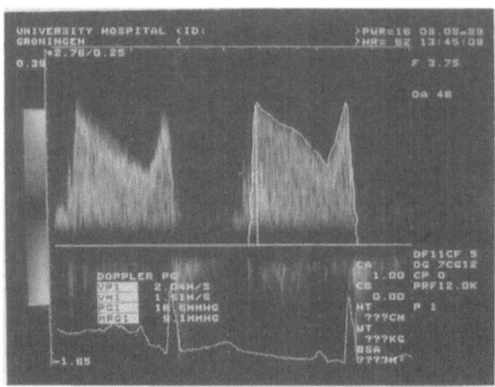

Fig. 134. Apical CW Doppler recording of mitral stenosis. From the traced signal a peak pressure difference (PG1) of 16.6 mm Hg is calculated and a mean pressure difference (MPG1) of 9.1 mm Hg. The $t^1/_2p$ is 168 ms, MVA 131 mm^2. The heart rate is 62 b/min.

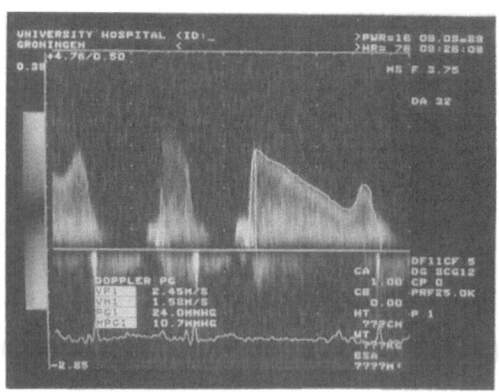

Fig. 135. Apical CW Doppler recording of mitral stenosis. PG1 is 24.0 mm Hg, MPG 10.7 mm Hg. The $t^1/_2p$ is 248 ms and MVA 88.7 mm^2. Note the small difference with the mean pressure difference of Fig. 8-134, but the large difference in mitral valve area. The heart rate is 76 b/min.

Since none of the methods mentioned are ideal, it is advisable to use at least two.

Further evaluation of the severity
Initially, a patient with mitral stenosis has complaints during physical exertion. Thus, complaints are related to the heart rate. Complaints are also quite subjective and patient expectations vary greatly. Thus, it is logical that, if complaints only exist during physical exertion, Doppler measurements should also be made during or immediately following physical exertion. The peak

pressure difference, measured just after physical exertion, is not predictable from the values at rest.

Under-estimation of the severity
Besides the causes mentioned earlier, Doppler measurements underestimate the severity of mitral stenosis if there is an angle between direction of flow and Doppler sound beam (angle). For the majority of patients the angle is too small to be important but for many patients this under-estimation is clinically significant.

With CW Doppler alone, the best signal is obtained from the apical view by recording and listening to the audio signal. The LV inflow is usually directed towards the LV lateral wall. With the transducer at the apex, there is often an angle; this angle cannot be made smaller as the transducer would have to be moved more to the left where lung tissue interferes with the echo and Doppler signals.

The angle can be visualized with color Doppler. Two conditions have to be fullfilled to calculate a correct angle.

Firstly, the color flow should originate from the mitral valve itself. If not, the angle may be under-estimated if the flow is curved (Fig. 8-136, 8-137, 8-138).

Secondly, with the point of inflow in the middle of the sector, and originating from the mitral ostium, the transducer should be rotated around its long axis in order to make the angle as large as possible (Fig. 8-139, 8-140). This is to include a possible angle between the flow direction and the sector plane. The CW line is positioned then through the mitral ostium and the flow velocity, corrected for the angle, is measured.

To be investigated in mitral stenosis
echocardiography:
- M-mode recording from the valve: anterior motion of the PML during diastole. Valve thickening? Calcifications? (long axis view)
- LV dimensions, description of the velocity of relaxation (long axis view)
- LA dimensions and contents (thrombi?) (long axis, apical view)
- RA dimensions (apical view)
- IVC diameters during respiration

Doppler:
- mitral insufficiency? (apical view)

color Doppler:
- (+CW) correction of measurements for the angle; peak- and mean pressure difference, $t^1/_2p$ value. Measurements at rest and following physical exertion (apical view)
- (+CW) peak pressure of the RV

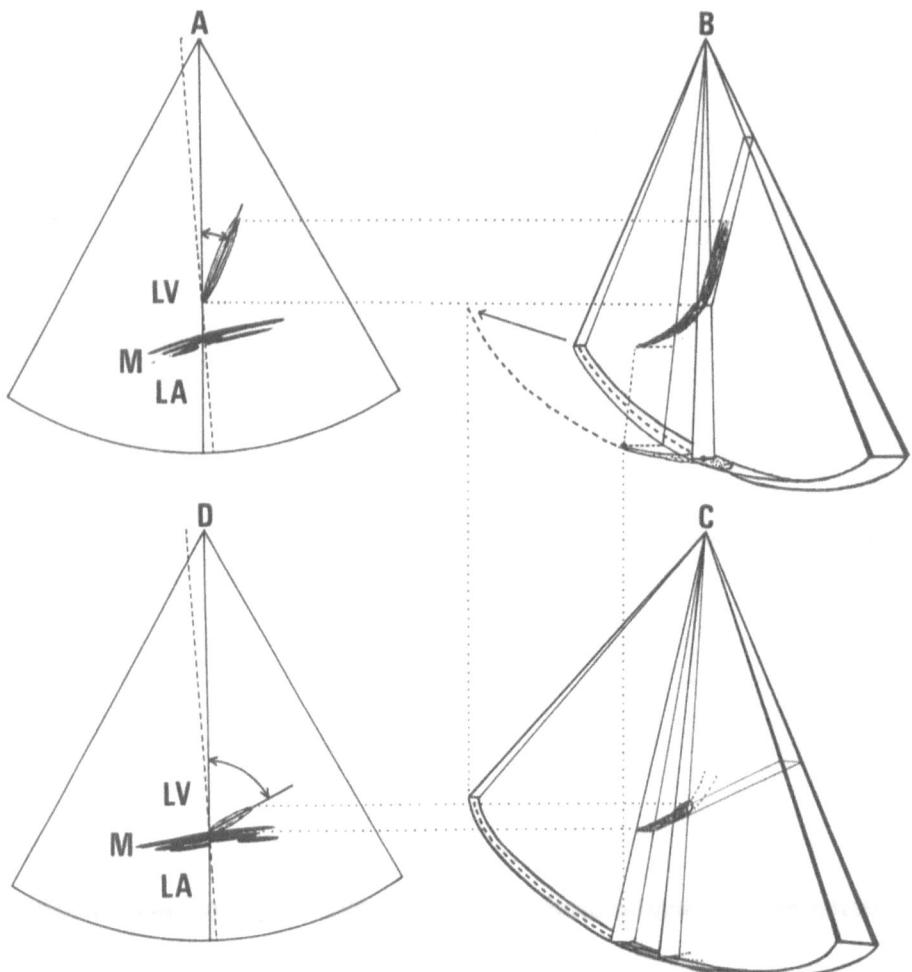

Fig. 8-136. Schematic apical color Doppler recording of mitral stenosis. At A the color flow does not originate from the mitral valve (M); there is only a small angle. The flow may be curved, as in B; in the example the transducer should be directed more to the left and rotated anticlockwise in order to let the color area start at the mitral ostium (C). This results in a sector image with a much larger and correct angle.

PULMONIC VALVE

The normal pulmonic valve

The echocardiographic evaluation of the pulmonic valve in the adult is difficult and often disappointing. From the short axis aortic view, the direction of the

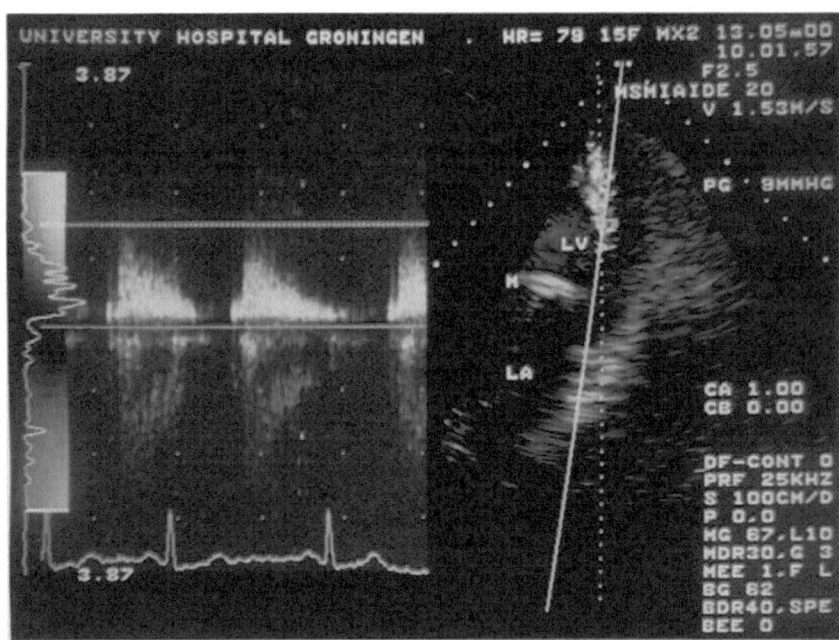

Fig. 8-137. Practical example of Fig. 8-136A. A peak pressure difference is measured of 9 mm Hg, heart rate 79 b/min.

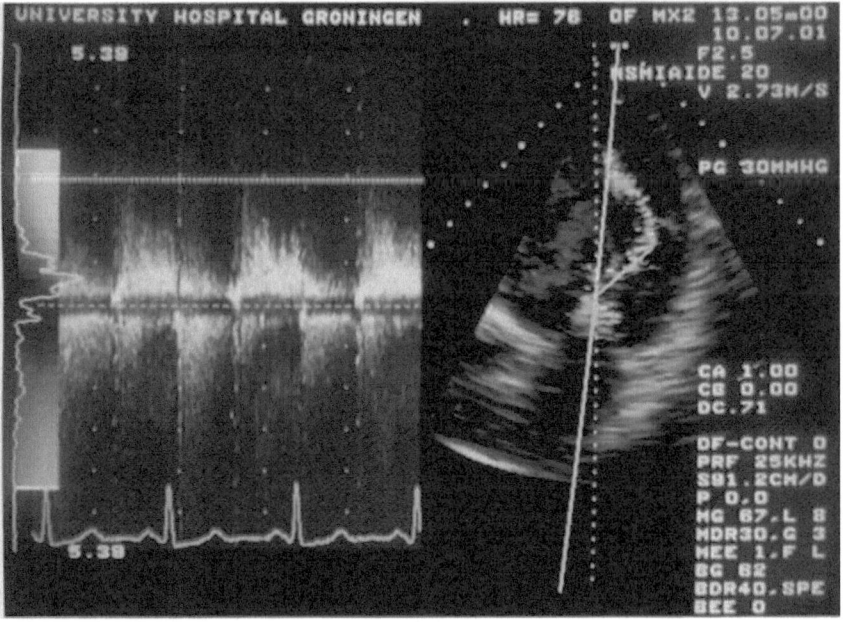

Fig. 8-138. Practical example of Fig. 8-136D from the same patient as Fig. 8-137. The transducer has been rotated and angled to let the color flow originate from the mitral valve. There appears to be an angle of 45° (DC 71); instead of a pressure difference of 9 mm Hg, it is -after correction for the angle) 30 mm Hg, heart rate 76 b/min, which correlated well with catheterization data.

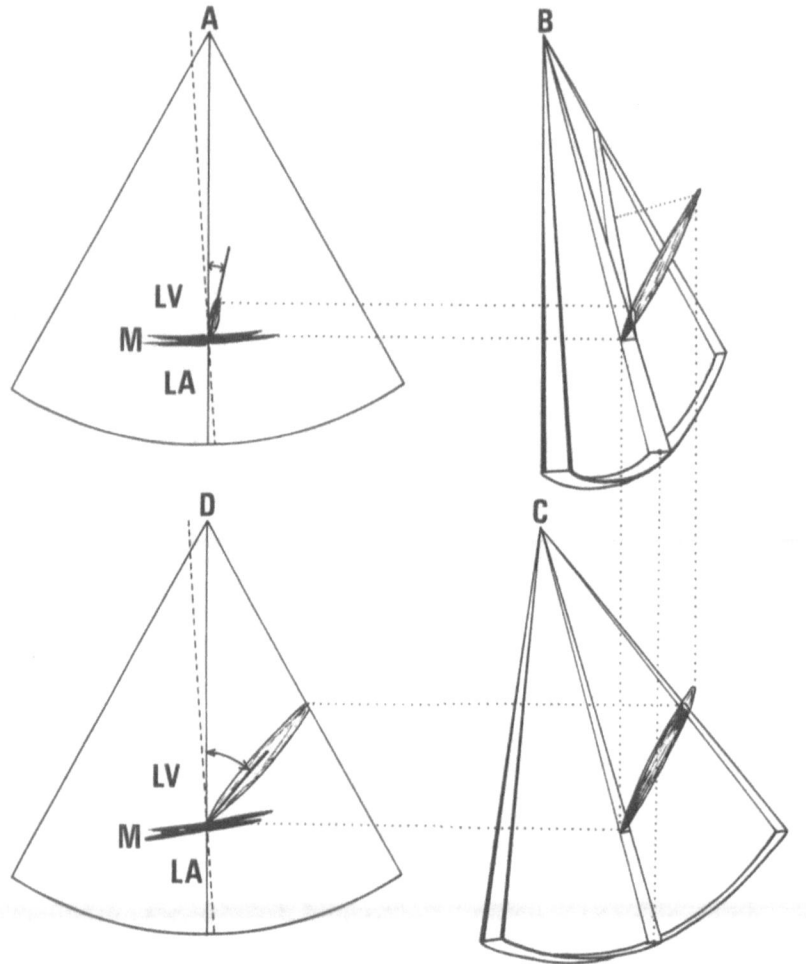

Fig. 8-139. Apical color Doppler signal of the mitral valve (M). Since there may be angle between the sector plane and the direction of flow (B), the transducer should be rotated around its long axis (C) to find the correct angle (D).

sound beam is in line with the main pulmonary artery. Echoes from the closed valve can usually be seen from only one of the three cusps. The opened valve is often not visible in the adult.

On the M-mode recording, the closure line is identified as a straight line during diastole. The atrial contraction is visible as a downward motion of 2-4 mm of the closure line. This is called the a-dip. If less than 2 mm or absent, pulmonary hypertension is likely to exist (Fig. 8-141). If the a-dip is more than 4 mm, pulmonic stenosis may be present. The a-dip is absent in atrial fibrillation.

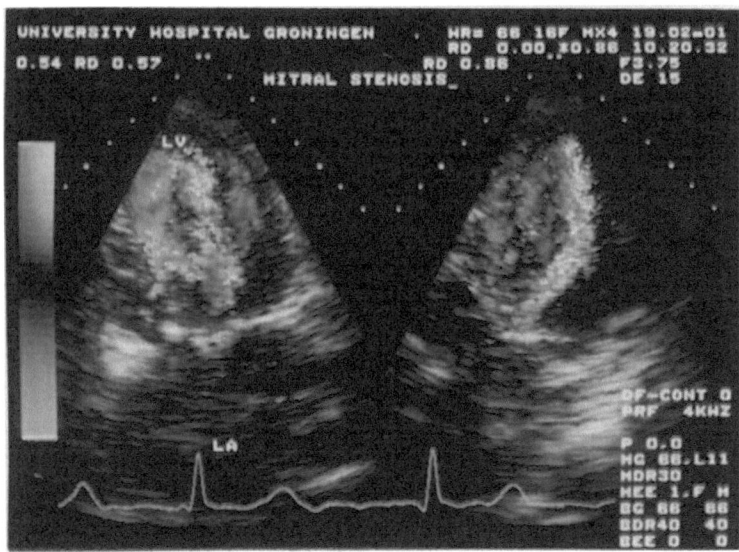

Fig. 8-140. Practical example of Fig. 8-139. On the left a standard 4-chamber view shows mitral stenosis flow directed without angle towards the transducer (Fig. 8-139A). After rotation an angle is found (Fig. 8-139D) for which measurements should be corrected.

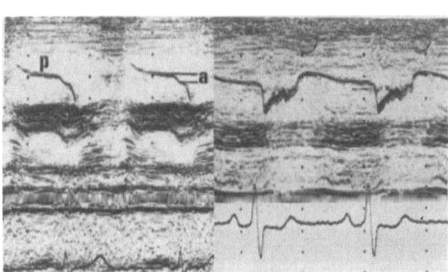

Fig. 8-141. Short axis aortic M-mode recording of a normal pulmonic valve (p) (left) and of the pulmonic valve in pulmonary hypertension. The normal valve shows an a-dip (a) of 3 mm as a result of atrial contraction. Usually, the a-dip is absent in pulmonary hypertension (right).

Doppler findings from the normal pulmonic valve are discussed in Chapter 7.

Pulmonic stenosis

Pulmonic stenosis is a congenital abnormality. Most patients are asymptomatic. In severe stenosis, dyspnea and fatigue at physical exertion are the most common symptoms. Exertional syncope is possible. Occasionally, angina-like chest pain is possible in very severe stenosis, caused by increased RV oxygen demands because of hypertrophy.

From the short axis aortic view, pulmonic stenosis can be suspected from the M-mode recording if the a-dip is more than 4 mm, e.g. 6-8 mm. On the other hand, pulmonic stenosis can be rather severe in the presence of a normal a-dip. The systolic pattern of the pulmonic valve on M-mode hardly has any value for the diagnosis of valvular pulmonic stenosis. From the long axis view, a para-doxical motion pattern of the IVS may be found, also in the absence of volume overload. The RV wall may be thickened.

The best position for Doppler examinations is the short axis aortic view where a parallel or nearly parallel alignment to flow is found. From the subcostal view, a recording of the Doppler signal is barely possible in adults.

Increased flow velocities may indicate pulmonic stenosis. They can also be caused by a left-to-right shunt or moderate to severe pulmonic insufficiency. The causes are differentiated by detecting these abnormalities and by the characteristic audio signals and flow velocity curves.

The maximal flow velocity can be found by recording the CW Doppler signal, and listening to the audio signal. The shape of the Doppler signal is the same as for aortic stenosis. The peak and mean systolic pressure differences can be calculated from this signal. Color Doppler is sometimes useful to provide spatial orientation of the jet. If turbulent flow is detected with color below the pulmonic valve in the RV, sub-valvular obstruction or the presence of a VSD should be suspected. This is discussed in Chapter 8, 'right ventricle')

If pulmonary hypertension is also present, the acceleration time is decreased (< 110 ms).

To be investigated in valvular pulmonic stenosis
echocardiography:
- depth of the a-dip (short axis aortic view)
- RV wall thickness (long axis view)
- septal motion. Paradoxical? (long axis view)
Doppler:
- pressure difference across the valve (with the heart rate)
- is there a 'stenotic' audio signal? Are there no superimposed signals, caused by sub-valvular pulmonic stenosis?
color Doppler:
- (+CW) is there an angle between direction of flow and CW sound beam? If so, the flow velocity should be corrected for this.
- is moderate or severe pulmonic insufficiency present?

To be excluded:
- sub-valvular pulmonic stenosis
- ASD
- VSD
- aortic stenosis

Sub-valvular pulmonic stenosis

As the consequences of sub-valvular pulmonic stenosis for hemodynamics are the same, the complaints are also the same as for valvular stenosis.

The echocardiographic and Doppler recordings in sub-valvular pulmonic stenosis are the best from the short axis aortic view. Sometimes, additional information is obtained with color Doppler from the apical view.

The M-mode aspect of the pulmonic valve in sub-valvular stenosis is typical and comparable with that from the aortic valve in sub-valvular aortic stenosis. During systole a coarse flutter is recorded, in severe sub-valvular stenosis accompanied by a mid- and/or late-systolic tendency to close.

The Doppler signal has a characteristic pattern. A superimposed flow is recorded of lower velocity with a late-systolic peak, representing the flow velocity in the RV outflow tract. With color, turbulent flow is recorded in the RV outflow tract (Fig. 8-38). This may also be caused by a VSD which has to be excluded.

When sub-valvular and valvular stenosis coexist, the infundibular flow signal is superimposed upon the pulmonary artery flow signal. The infundibular flow has a late-systolic peak, as it is a dynamic obstruction. If the flow velocity through the infundibulum is increased, it has to be included in the measurement of the valvular peak velocity. If it is not included, the severity of pulmonic stenosis is over-estimated.

The differentiation between a low positioned sub-valvular stenosis and a double chambered RV may be difficult (Fig. 8-38, 8-39). The short axis aortic view and the apical view in combination with color Doppler are then helpful.

To be investigated in sub-valvular pulmonic stenosis
- the same questions as in valvular pulmonic stenosis

To be excluded:
- valvular pulmonic stenosis
- double chambered RV
- ASD
- VSD
- aortic stenosis

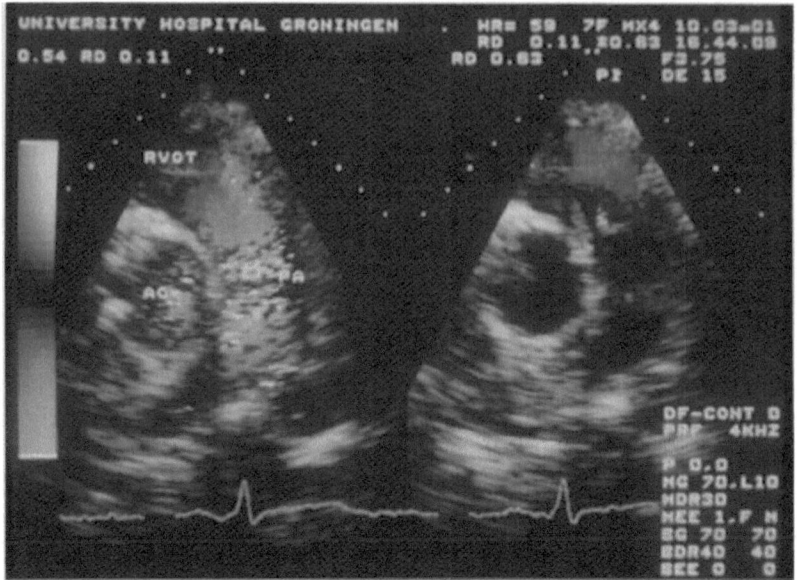

Fig. 8-142. Short axis aortic color Doppler of a normal pulmonic valve. On the right of the aorta, below the RV outflow tract (RVOT), blue colors show the systolic flow towards the pulmonary artery (PA). The red colors show the position of the pulmonic valve. Below the main pulmonary artery and behind the aorta, the right pulmonary artery is seen as a black area; the other black area on the right is the left pulmonary artery. During diastole (right) the pulmonic valve is closed, but two small red flames show physiological pulmonic insufficiency, one in the centre of the valve and a larger one between two valve leaflets against the pulmonic ring.

Pulmonic insufficiency

Isolated pulmonic insufficiency may be tolerated for many years without complaints. If complicated by pulmonary hypertension, fatigue and dyspnea may be severe and cyanosis may be present.

Physiological pulmonic insufficiency is rather common. There is some relationship between the intensity of the Doppler signal and the severity of the insufficiency. The intensity of the regurgitant flow should then be compared with that from the forward flow. Also, in mild insufficiency, the flow is often difficult to detect in very early diastole.

The intensity of color flow can be helpful in the differentiation between mild, moderate and severe insufficiency (Fig. 8-142).

Severe pulmonic insufficiency is found in endocarditis of the pulmonic valve. This is a rather rare condition. The valve is thickened then, with a good motion pattern. Often, a diastolic flutter can be recorded.

The flow velocity of pulmonic insufficiency can be used to determine whether or not the diastolic pressure in the pulmonary artery is increased. A flow velocity greater than 1.7 m/s is indicative for the presence of increased diastolic pulmonary artery pressure.

To be investigated in pulmonic insufficiency
echocardiography:
– diastolic flutter of the valve (short axis aortic view)
Doppler:
– is insufficiency difficult or easy to find? (short axis aortic view)
– is flow velocity increased (increased diastolic pulmonary artery pressure)?
color Doppler:
– is the color area deep in the RV?
– (+CW) RV peak pressure measured from tricuspid insufficiency

To be excluded:
– aortic insufficiency

THE TRICUSPID VALVE

The normal tricuspid valve

The M-mode recording and the flow velocity pattern of the tricuspid valve resemble that of the mitral valve. For the descriptions, we refer to Chapter 8, 'mitral valve'.

Tricuspid stenosis

Isolated tricuspid stenosis is a rare abnormality. Usually, tricuspid stenosis is found in combination with mitral stenosis. Tricuspid stenosis may also be present in the carcinoid syndrome. This syndrome is characterized by cutaneous flushing, diarrhea and bronchial obstruction, and is caused by the release of serotonin by carcinoid tumors. Endocardial plaques can be found, composed of a unique type of fibrous tissue. Tricuspid and pulmonic valves are distorted and thickened (Fig. 8-143). In carcinoid syndrome tricuspid stenosis is usually combined with severe tricuspid insufficiency (Fig. 8-144).

Complaints in tricuspid stenosis are related to impaired RV filling: dyspnea on exertion, which may be severe also at rest. Abdominal pain is possible because of liver enlargement. Peripheral edema can be found.

The best transducer positions for examining the tricuspid valve are the short axis aortic view and the apical view. The subcostal view may also be useful. A

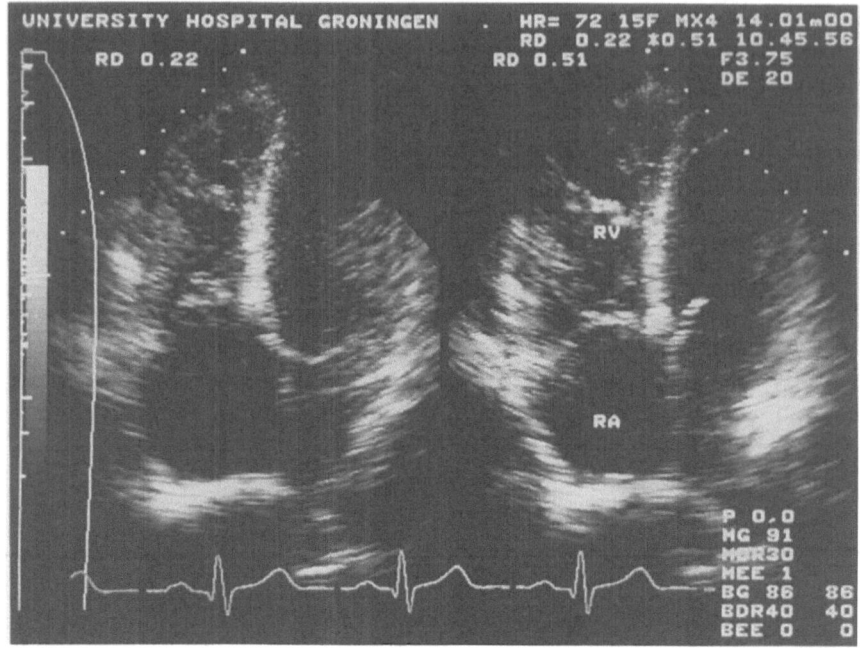

Fig. 8-143. Apical view of carcinoid syndrome. The structures in the RV are accentuated and thickened. The echoes from the tricuspid area barely change in position between systole (left) and diastole, indicating a stiff, possibly stenotic tricuspid valve. The RA is enlarged.

typical doming can be found of the tricuspid valve in tricuspid stenosis. The leaflets may be thickened. The aspect on M-mode and the Doppler signal resemble that from mitral stenosis. With Doppler, peak pressures can be measured to evaluate the severity. Also, mean pressure differences and t^1/$_2$p values can be calculated as described in Chapter 8, 'mitral valve'.

To be investigated in tricuspid stenosis
echocardiography:
– M-mode recording (apical, short axis aortic, subcostal view)
– RA dimension (apical, short axis aortic, subcostal view)
– dimensions of the IVC during respiration
color Doppler:
– (+CW) angle-corrected pressure difference across the valve

Tricuspid insufficiency

Physiological tricuspid insufficiency is common. Only severe tricuspid in-

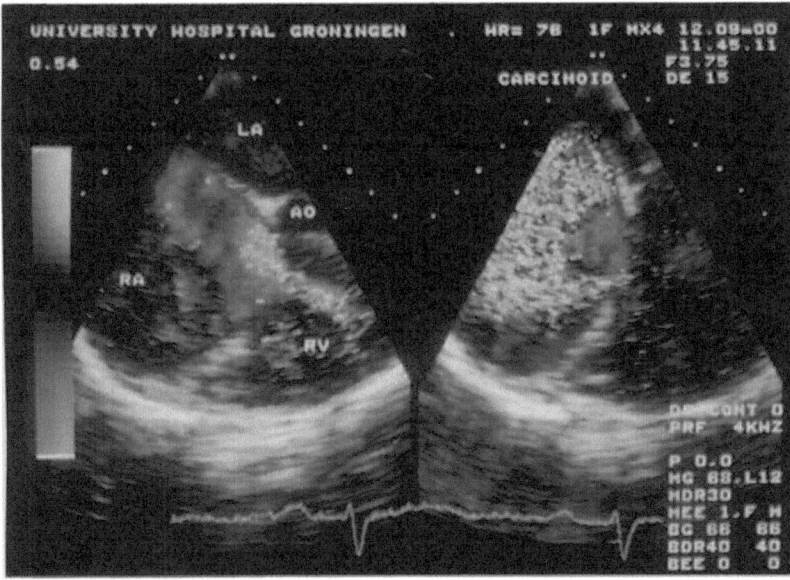

Fig. 8-144. TEE recording of carcinoid syndrome. The visible part of the tricuspid valve is thickened and hardly moves. During diastole (left) a turbulent inflow into the RV suggests tricuspid stenosis, but it may also be caused by massive tricuspid insufficiency. This is visible from the systolic frame where the RA is almost filled with turbulent colors. AO = aorta.

sufficiency may result in dyspnea on exertion or also at rest. The central venous pressure is increased, which is measurable from distended neck veins. The liver is enlarged, which may be painful. Peripheral edema is found. The liver may be damaged with impairment of liver functions.

Usually, the M-mode recording from a tricuspid valve with insufficiency is the same as from a competent valve. Occasionally, tricuspid valve prolapse is found or a post-traumatic chordal rupture (Fig. 8-145).

Mostly, tricuspid insufficiency is secondary to mitral valve disease. The pulmonary artery and RV pressures increase. The RV enlarges with also dilatation of the tricuspid ring, resulting in tricuspid insufficiency.

If color Doppler is not available, contrast echocardiography may be helpful for the detection of tricuspid insufficiency (Chapter 4). However, the severity is difficult to detect with this method.

Transducer positions for the Doppler examination of tricuspid insufficiency are the short axis aortic, the apical, the subcostal and the IVC views. As calculation of the RV peak pressure also can be performed from the peak flow velocities of tricuspid insufficiency, the short axis aortic view is the best one, as correction for an angle is easier there: rather often the quality of the colors is poor from the apical view. If flow velocities can only be measured from the

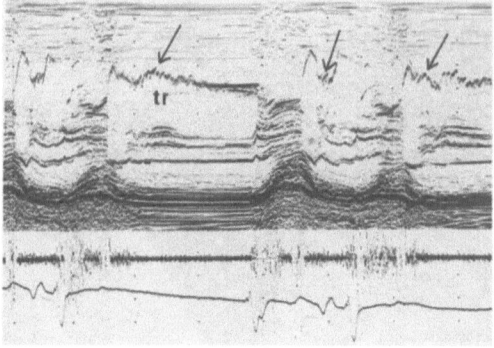

Fig. 8-145. M-mode recording of a post-traumatic chordal rupture of the tricuspid valve (tr). As in chordal rupture of the mitral valve, a coarse, irregular flutter is recorded from the valve leaflets (arrows).

subcostal position, visualization of the direction of flow with color is also necessary to correct the measurement for the angle. This is especially the case in patients with emphysema in whom a parasternal or apical view cannot be obtained. There is much interest in the presence and the severity of pulmonary hypertension in these patients.

The CW signal from tricuspid insufficiency very much resembles that from mitral insufficiency (Fig. 7-3, 8-106). For measurements of RV peak pressures from the CW signal we refer to Chapter 8 'right ventricle'.

With color Doppler, the color area could be used to express the severity, but this method has the same problems as mentioned with mitral insufficiency.

The change in diameter of the IVC is helpful in evaluating tricuspid in-

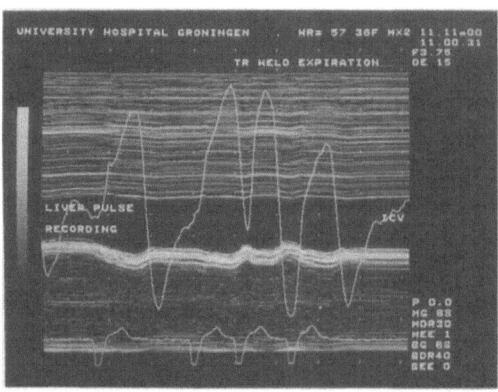

Fig. 8-146. M-mode recording of the IVC and liver pulse recording in tricuspid insufficiency. Dilatation of the vessel (filling from the RA) is seen during ventricular systole which coincides with a positive deflection of the liver pulse recording.

sufficiency (Fig. 8-146). In the normal heart the IVC collapses during ventricular systole, but in tricuspid insufficiency it dilates. This is also seen from the liver pulse recording.

Color Doppler flow imaging of liver veins in tricuspid insufficiency from the IVC position shows a systolic red color caused by backflow into the liver. This is a good hallmark for the presence of insufficiency. To determine the severity of tricuspid insufficiency the liver pulse recording still seems to be the best. If the liver pulse recording is positive during systole (S-wave) tricuspid insufficiency is judged to be severe. Tricuspid valve repair is advisable then, when the mitral valve is replaced for mitral stenosis and/or insufficiency.

To be investigated in tricuspid insufficiency
echocardiography:
– M-mode recording (apical, short axis aortic, subcostal view)
– RA dimension (apical, short axis aortic, subcostal view)
– dimensions of the ICV during respiration
color Doppler:
– (+CW) angle-corrected systolic pressure difference across the valve (RV peak pressure) (short axis aortic, apical and/or subcostal view)
– color area?
pulse recording:
– S-wave (liver pulse)

PROSTHETIC VALVES

Evaluation of prosthetic valve function

The echocardiographic evaluation of prosthetic valves is difficult. This is partly caused by the materials from which the valves are made. The velocity of ultrasound in cardiac muscle and blood differs from the velocity through metals and plastics. Also, reverberations are common in prosthetic valves, shielding the area behind them.

Tilting disc prosthetic valves, bileaflet prostheses with two tilting discs and bioprosthetic valves are most commonly implanted.

The echocardiographic aspect of the Björk-Shiley valve depends somewhat on the surgical insertion. Impairment of opening by thrombi is difficult to evaluate. The thrombus itself may be shielded. It is not possible to measure the excursion of the disc with echocardiography. Occasionally, in very severe obstruction, poor excursions are obvious. In that case, the effects of the obstruction on the systolic and diastolic ventricular diameters can also be seen. On the M-mode recording, the E point should be sharply pointed (Fig. 8-147).

184

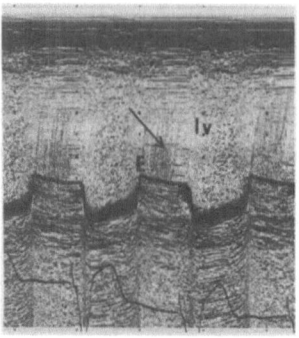

Fig. 8-147. Normal Björk-Shiley mitral prosthesis from the apical view. E is sharply pointed. Spontaneous contrast is also recorded (arrow).

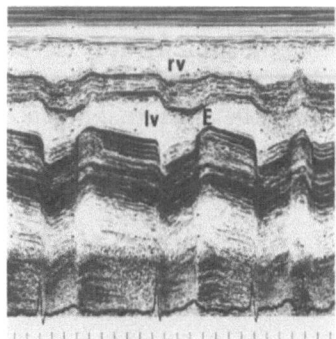

Fig. 8-148. Apical Björk-Shiley prosthesis with severe paravalvular insufficiency. This is suggested by the rounded E point. Paravalvular insufficiency was confirmed at surgery.

A rounded E point may be found in severe paravalvular insufficiency (Fig. 8-148) and also in valvular obstruction.

The echocardiographic evaluation of the St. Jude prosthetic valve is not as simple as would be expected. Various recordings are possible, depending on transducer position and on surgical insertion.

The bioprosthetic valves are easier to evaluate. The motion pattern of these valves can easily be evaluated. The stents are more echogenic than in normal valve rings.

Doppler echocardiography is extremely helpful in assessing the function of prosthetic valves. The transvalvular pressure difference can be measured, as well as the presence of paravalvular and valvular insufficiency. The most reliable pressure measurements are obtained from bioprostheses and St. Jude valves, as they have a central opening. It is very likely that, from the apical view, the flow is directed straight towards or away from the transducer for both left sided valves, which results in a correct measurement. In aortic and mitral Björk-Shiley valves, under-estimation of the pressure difference is logic, as the disc does not open 90° and the flow is not directed towards the transducer. Color Doppler is then necessary for establishing the angle between directions of flow and CW Doppler sound beam. Irrespective of the directions of flow however, is the steepness of the downward slope of the CW signal in early diastole in mitral valves.

The direction of flow through a Björk-Shiley prosthesis depends somewhat on the surgical insertion. In the long axis view the flow through a Björk-Shiley mitral prosthesis is often directed somewhat to the IVS (Fig. 8-149). In several patients an abnormal direction of flow can be found almost perpendicular to the IVS. This suggests obstruction of the valve by a thrombus mass or endothelial proliferation. Mitral inflow with too sharp an angle of inflow can also been seen from the apical view if obstruction is present. With color, from several views, only one color flow area instead of two are found which is also suggestive for inflow obstruction.

Over-estimation of the peak pressure difference across a prosthetic valve is not uncommon. From St Jude valves, Duromedics valves as well as from Björk-Shiley valves flow velocities corresponding with pressure differences of 30-35 mm Hg at normal heart rates have often been found. Those signals are usually weak, but have a typical high pitched audio signal. They obviously originated from the area of the prosthetic ring. Pressure differences of about 8 mm Hg can also be found from the same valves, with better signals. At simultaneous cardiac catheterization, this figure is usually confirmed.

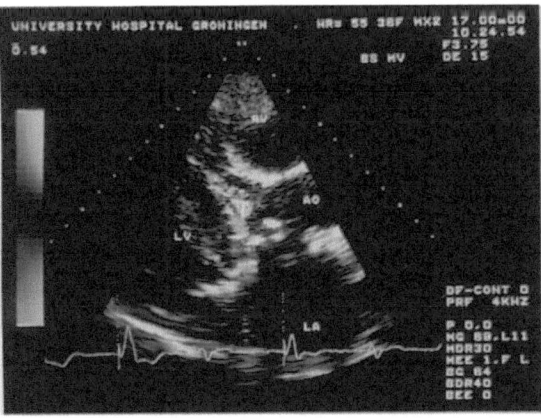

Fig. 8-149. Left parasternal recording of a Björk-Shiley mitral prosthesis. The direction of flow almost perpendicular to the IVS almost proves impaired valve opening by a thrombus mass, which was confirmed at surgery.

Regurgitation through or along a prosthetic valve can rather often be found. Regurgitation from an aortic valve prosthesis is diagnosed from the apical and parasternal views, as shielding is then in the other direction. Regurgitation from a mitral prosthesis is technically more difficult to evaluate. Sometimes it can be diagnosed with Doppler from the apical view: with CW a signal away from the transducer can be recorded. Color Doppler is most helpful for the detection of (para)valvular mitral insufficiency: a systolic blue color can be found in the LV that ends in the region of the the prosthetic valve ring; the color has to be differentiated from the normal blue color, directed towards the aortic area: the color towards the aorta starts later in systole. TEE is superior to these transducer positions and mitral paravalvular or valvular insufficiency can be clearly seen without the shielding problem. Even very small insufficiencies can be diagnosed (Fig. 8-150). Also, abnormal motion patterns and other problems of prosthetic valves can be evaluated very well with TEE (Fig. 8-151).

Endocarditis and prosthetic valves

The detection of prosthetic valve endocarditis is a major problem. Vegetations

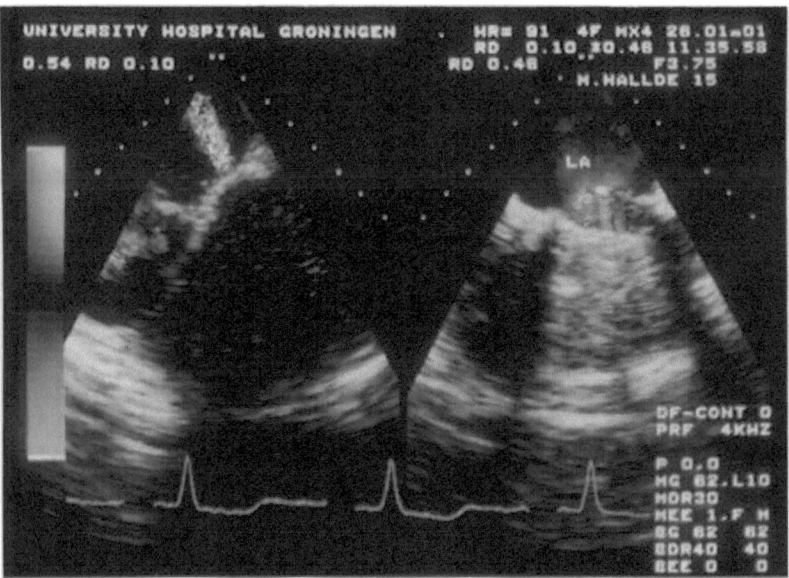

Fig. 8-150. TEE of a Medtronic Hall mitral prosthesis. During diastole (right) blue colors with aliasing show a normal inflow in the LV. During ventricular systole a small area of turbulent colors in the LA indicate paravalvular insufficiency (left).

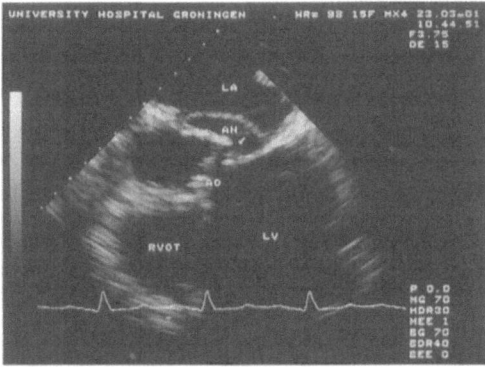

Fig. 8-151. TEE of a mechanical aortic valve prosthesis. Aortic insufficiency was audible. With TEE a dissection-like aneurysmatic dilatation of the aortic root is found (AN) with a small connection to the LV outflow tract (arrow). AO = position of aortic valve prosthesis.

are easily masked by the echogenic prosthetic valves and by shielding but the problem of shielding can be excluded by using TEE. Fig. 8-152 illustrates an impaired motion of a Björk-Shiley aortic prosthesis by a vegetation in the LV outflow tract. In endocarditis of an aortic valve prosthesis, paravalvular abscesses may be found.

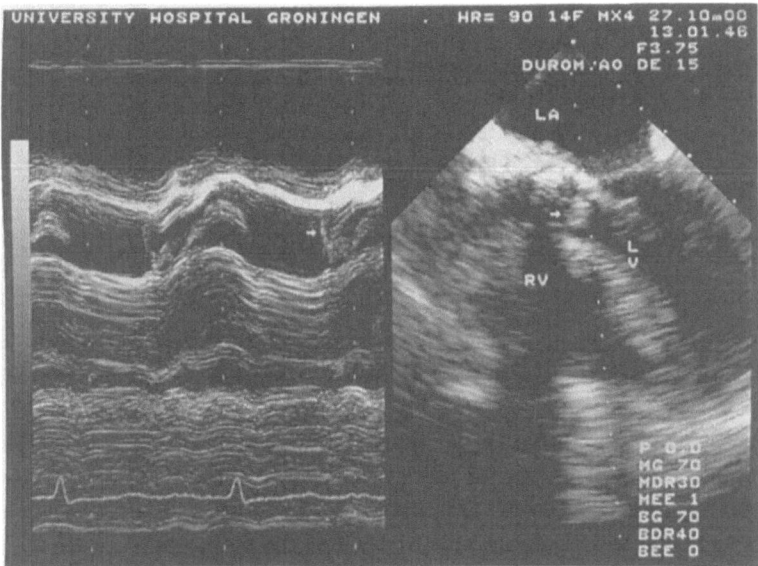

Fig. 8-152. TEE of a Duromedics aortic prosthesis with aortic insufficiency. An echogenic mobile structure is found in the LV outflow tract (arrows) that impairs normal closure of the prosthesis. At surgery a vegetation was removed.

For the evaluation of prosthetic valve endocarditis all possible transducer positions should be used, especially TEE which is indispensable in this respect.

THORACIC AORTA

Coarctation

Coarctation of the aorta is a congenital stenosis of the distal aortic arch or of the descending aorta. Usually, the constriction of the aorta is found just distal to the left subclavian artery.

In severe coarctation, the blood pressure measured in the upper part of the body is increased and higher than the blood pressure in the lower part. Because of the high blood pressure in the upper part of the body, the patient may complain of headache and dizziness. The low blood pressure in the legs may cause cold feet. Pulsations of the femoral artery are poor. A murmur can be heard at the second intercostal space on the left and on the back. The murmur starts a short time after aortic valve opening and ends after the aortic closure sound.

In combination with coarctation, deformation of the aortic valve may be present, such as a bicuspid valve. Aortic insufficiency and/or aortic stenosis may be present. A VSD may also be found.

As coarctation is a LV pressure overload, the same features can be found from the LV as are found in hypertension.

Trans-thoracic echocardiography is not very useful for the detection of coarctation. From the suprasternal view, the sound beams are parallel to the smooth walls of the aorta. This makes reliable visualization of a coarctation difficult. Also, a false positive diagnosis can be made, caused by buckling of the descending aorta.

TEE is more helpful than TTE for the visualization of coarctation.

The hemodynamic significance of a coarcation is measured with CW from the suprasternal view. The pressure proximal to the coarctation is measured and should be subtracted from the pressure, derived from the peak velocity (Fig. 8-153).

The effects of coarctation on the heart are found from the parasternal view: a thickened LV wall, in severe cases dilatation of the LV. The LA may be enlarged by an increased LVEDP.

The aortic valve is evaluated for the number of cusps and the presence of aortic insufficiency and/or stenosis. A coarctation masks (the severity of) aortic valve stenosis: it is under-estimated with Doppler. Consequently, the echocardiographic aspect of the aortic valve is important.

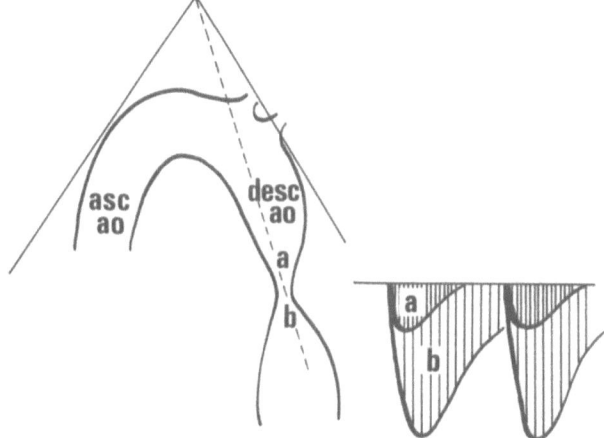

Fig. 8-153. Schematic representation of coarctation. The CW signal through the descending aorta (desc ao) shows two intensities: 'a' is the flow velocity proximal to the coarctation and 'b' distal to the coarctation. For calculating the pressure gradient across the coarctation 'a' should be subtracted from 'b'. asc ao = ascending aorta.

To be investigated in coarctation

echocardiography:
– visualization of the coarctation (suprasternal view, TEE)
– LV wall thickness (parasternal view)
– LV diameters (parasternal view)
– LA diameters (parasternal, apical view)
– aspect of the aortic valve (short axis aortic view)

Doppler:
– pressure difference across the coarctation (suprasternal view)
– pressure difference across the aortic valve
– aortic insufficiency

color Doppler:
– visualization of the flow through the coarctation
– estimation of the severity of aortic insufficiency

pulse recording:
– a/H ratio (ACG)

Dissection

Dissection of the aorta (dissecting aneurysm) is caused by a tear in the aortic wall. The blood, entering the aortic wall, destroys the media and strips the intima from the adventitia for variable distances. This can happen at various

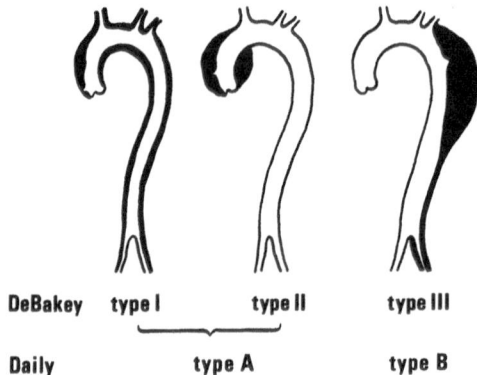

Fig. 8-154. Schematic representation of types of dissection according to DeBakey and according to Daily.

levels (Fig. 8-154). According to DeBakey there are three types of dissection, type I, II and III. Daily made a division into two types A and B, from wich type A includes DeBakey type I and II.

The complaints can mimic the complaints from myocardial infarction: a typical precordial chest pain may be present, but more often the pain is located in the neck or in the back, between the scapulae.

The echocardiographic diagnosis is definite when a true lumen is found, separated from a false lumen by an intimal flap. Sometimes, from the left parasternal transducer position, a dilatation of the ascending aorta with an intimal flap are found just above the aortic valve area together with aortic insufficiency. Sometimes the intimal flap can also be found from the suprasternal position (Fig. 8-155, 8-156).

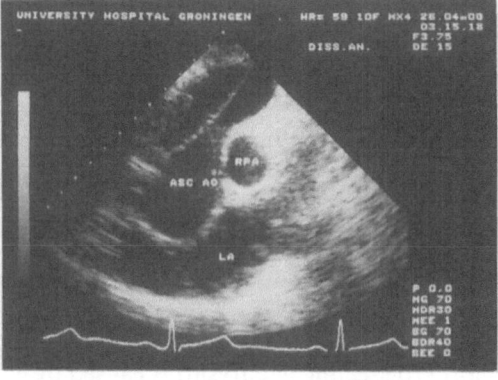

Fig. 8-155. Suprasternal recording of a dissection. An intimal flap is recorded in the middle of the ascending aorta (ASC AO). RPA = right pulmonary artery.

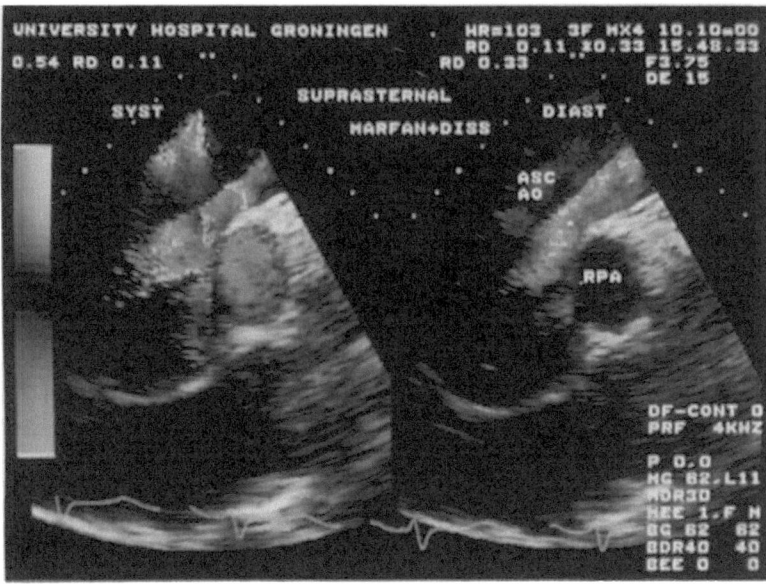

Fig. 8-156. Suprasternal recording of a dissection. During systole two areas of red colors with aliasing divide the ascending aorta (ASC AO) into two parts. During diastole the blue color in the lower part proves aortic regurgitation. RPA = right pulmonary artery.

The ideal method for detection or exclusion of aortic dissection is TEE. The ultrasound then hits the walls of the descending aorta (Fig. 8-157) and the first part of the ascending aorta (Fig. 8-158, 8-159) perpendicularly, resulting in magnificant echocardiographic images. With color Doppler a distinction can be made between the false and the true lumen.

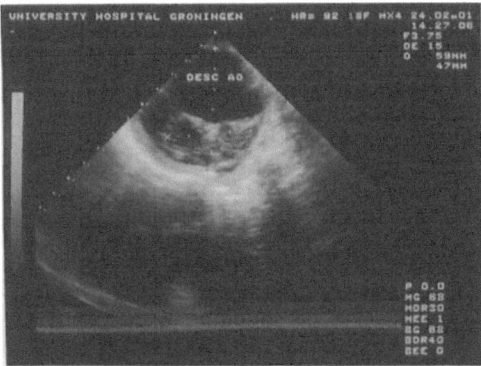

Fig. 8-157. Transverse section of the descending thoracic aorta with a dissection and a thrombus mass in the false lumen. From this frame only a mass can be identified (thrombus? plaque?) but the dissection was proven at autopsy.

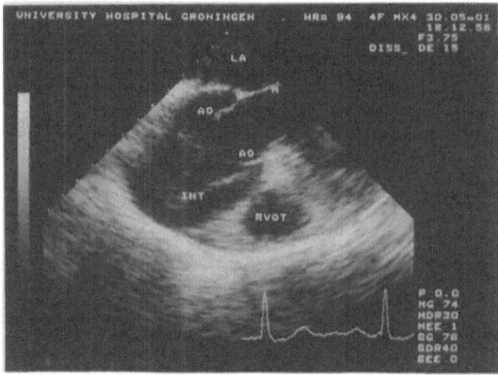

Fig. 8-158. TEE of dissection at the level of the aortic valve. Two of the three aortic cusps (AO) are visible in a widened aortic ring. Several intima layers (INT) prove dissection.

To be investigated in dissection of the aorta
echocardiography:
– dilatation of part of the aorta (long axis, suprasternal view)
– visualization of the intimal flap (long axis, suprasternal view)

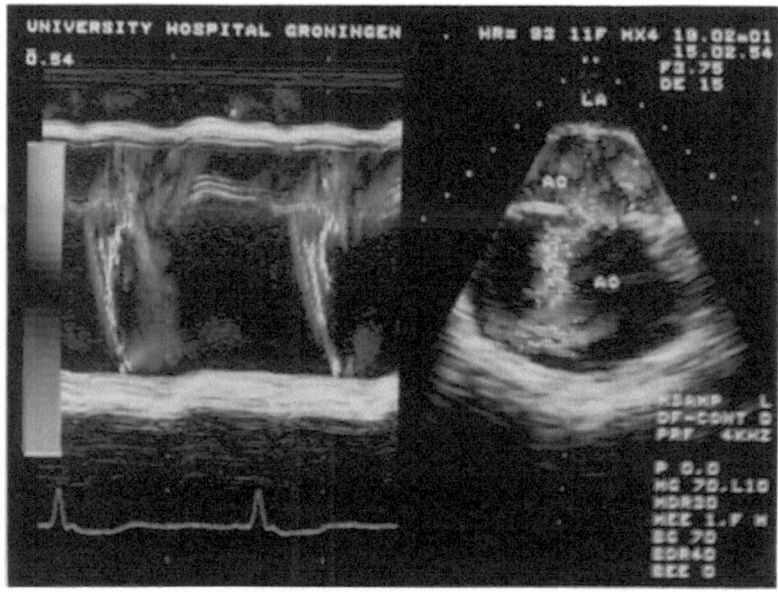

Fig. 8-159. TEE a few centimeters above the aortic valve. The ascending aorta is widened and divided into two parts (AO,AO) by a membrane. Through a hole in the membrane turbulent colors show a flow from the true lumen (the upper one) to the false lumen.

Doppler:
– aortic insufficiency (long axis, apical view)
color Doppler:
– identification of false and true lumen
TEE:
– same questions as above, but also the extent of the dissection

ENDOCARDITIS

Endocarditis is usually found in the left heart as pressure differences across valves are greater there than in the right heart; valve 'injury' occurs more readily from mitral- and aortic insufficiency than from pulmonic- and tricuspid insufficiency. A common cause for endocarditis of the left heart is a dental extraction or other dental manipulations but often a cause cannot be found. Endocarditis of the right heart may be caused by the presence of an intracardiac catheter for a longer time. It can also be found in drug addicts, caused by contaminated drugs ore needles.

Vegetations may be present, consisting of blood components and often also bacteria. The size of vegetations varies from less than a millimeter to several centimeters. The inflammation also causes weakening of the structures of the heart, especially the heart valves. Valve rupture or perforation is a well known major complication.

Usually, patients with 'acute' endocarditis are very ill. The severity of endocarditis is also determined by the degree of destruction in the heart and thus by the hemodynamic state of the patient.

Echocardiography can be very helpful in establishing the diagnosis. If fresh vegetations are found, they prove endocarditis. On the other hand, if vegetations cannot be found, endocarditis can still be present since very small vegetations are not detected due to resolution problems.

Vegetations are recognized on the echocardiogram as bright, local thickenings at the leading edges of valves. Usually they are located on the low pressure side of an insufficient valve, in the presence of a normal motion pattern of that valve. A high mobility of such echoes supports the diagnosis of vegetations. If the motion pattern is impaired, together with local valve thickenings, vegetations can barely be differentiated from calcifications. Consequently, vegetations on calcified valves are difficult or impossible to diagnose.

The detection and recognition of vegetations depend on many factors, such as the picture quality and the size of the vegetations. Especially very small vegetations cannot be detected with echocardiography. As resolution is better with high frequency transducers, TEE is superior to TTE for evaluating vegetations and ruptures of mitral and aortic valves.

The findings of endocarditis are discussed in the Chapters on the valves concerned, VSD and prosthetic valves.

Illustrations of endocarditis of the aortic valve are: Fig. 8-82, 8-83, 8-84, 8-96, 8-97.

Illustrations of endocarditis of the mitral valve are: Fig. 8-119 to 8-126, 8-152.

To be investigated in endocarditis
echocardiography:
– local thickenings at the leading edges of valves (all possible views)
– normal valve motion or calcifications?
– valve insufficiencies?
– valve perforation?
Doppler:
– valve insufficiencies?
color:
– color area? Severity of valve insufficiency?
TEE:
– same questions as mentioned above.

Note: An echocardiograph is not a microscope. If echo-masses are found as described earlier, they only give strong suspicion of vegetations. They have to be differentiated from calcifications, thrombus masses and myxoma's.

Note: if vegetations are not found, the answer to the question 'Is there endocarditis?' should be at least: 'Vegetations have not been found which does not exclude endocarditis at all.' This suggests that the question should be put differently: 'Are there echoes, suspicious for valve vegetations?'.

PERICARDIAL DISEASES

Pericardial effusion

Some pericardial fluid is always present in the normal pericardial cavity. This can often be seen on the echocardiogram as an echo-free space that is only present during ventricular systole. During diastole, the epi- and pericardium are seen as a single layer. Usually, such echo-free spaces are found behind the left ventricle. Very often, especially in obese patients, a space can also be found in the pericardial cavity in front of the right ventricle. This space is not completely echo-free. A few echoes of low density in that region are usually caused by pericardial fat.

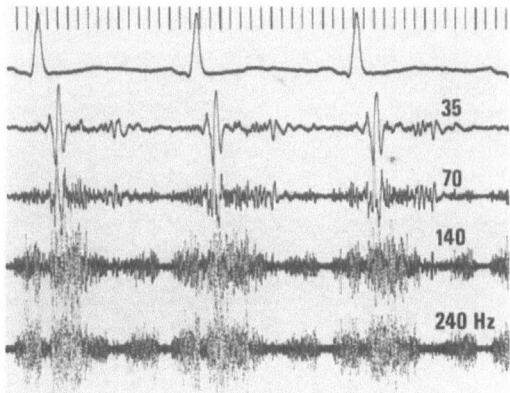

Fig. 8-160. Pericardial friction rub recorded on the 4th rib at the left side of the sternum. During one cardiac cycle a number of mid- and high frequency murmurs can be heard, independent of respiration, but sometimes dependent on the patient's position.

The volume of pericardial effusion is judged to be abnormal if an echo-free space is found between epi- and pericardium during systole as well as during diastole.

Pericardial effusion is found accidently or was suspected before echocardiography. The reason for suspecting effusion may have been the size and shape of the heart shadow on the chest X-ray, the presence of a pericardial friction rub or specific clinical findings.

Causes for pericardial effusion are pericarditis, bleeding after surgery and also neoplastic masses.

If a pericardial friction rub (Fig. 8-160) is heard, one should be aware of the fact that this does not necessarily mean that there is only a small amount of effusion, just enough to keep contact between epi- and pericardium. Classical friction rubs may be heard in the presence of $1^1/_2$ liters of pericardial fluid. The rub is explained by unequally divided pericardial effusion, with local contacts between epi- and pericardium. Unequal division of pericardial effusion is demonstrated in Fig. 8-161.

Pericardial effusion is not necessarily accompanied by complaints. Often, more than the 'physiologic' amount is found, whereas the echocardiographic examination was requested for other reasons. In case of pericarditis, fever is present and pain in the chest may be reported, sometimes resembling the pain caused by myocardial infarction. The severity of the pain depends on the patient's position. Patients with severe renal function disturbances usually have some pericardial effusion without pain.

If there is a large volume of pericardial effusion, the patient may be dyspnoic, caused by a filling problem of the heart. This situation is called tampo-

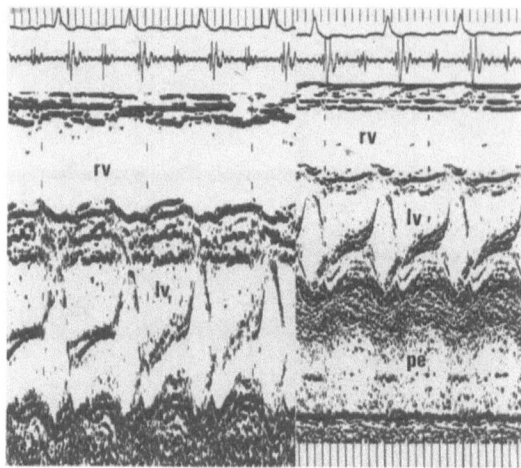

Fig. 8-161. Left parasternal recordings of pericardial effusion (pe). The left panel illustrates the importance of starting an examination with sufficient depth: there seems to be nothing abnormal behind the LV. However, the right panel with more depth shows much pericardial effusion behind the LV with echoes, suspicious for fibrin, against the epicardium. The presence of fibrin was confirmed at surgery, as was 900 cc pericardial effusion.

nade. In tamponade there is often so much pericardial effusion that the heart 'hangs' on the large vessels. Consequently, during contraction the whole heart moves to and fro during the cardiac cycle. This is called a 'swinging heart' (Fig. 8-162).

Extension of the whole heart, necessary during inspiration, is no longer possible in tamponade. However, during inspiration, the RA and RV volumes have to increase. As extension of the total heart is not possible, the RV volume

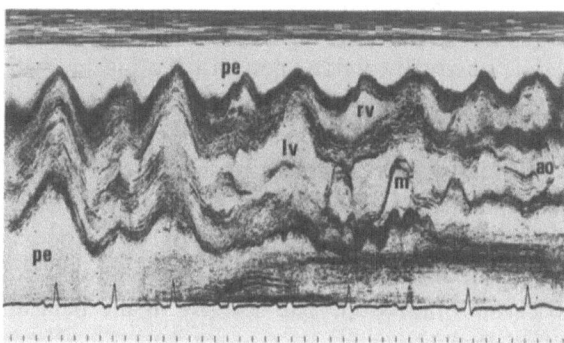

Fig. 8-162. Left parasternal M-mode sweep from the apex to the aorta in the presence of much pericardial effusion (pe). The aorta (ao) and surrounding structures are rather stable, but the heart shows the typical 'swinging heart'. m = mitral valve.

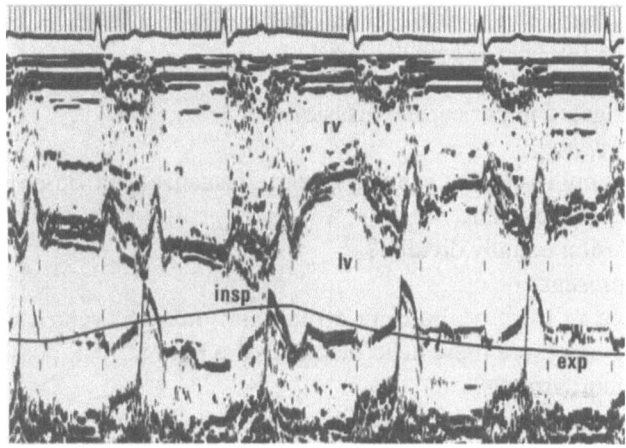

Fig. 8-163. Left parasternal M-mode recording at a paper speed of 25 mm/sec of constrictive pericarditis. The anteroposterior diameter of the whole heart is the same during this recording, but at inspiration the RV diameter increases (gray), resulting in a decreasing volume of the LV.

can only increase if the LV volume decreases. The same mechanism is also found in constrictive pericarditis. It can be visualized on the M-mode recording as a displacement of the IVS towards the LVPW during inspiration (Fig. 8-163). This phenomenon explains why the normal decrease of the systolic bloodpressure during inspiration (< 6 mm Hg) is greater in these patients (10-30 mm Hg).

These symptoms and findings in physical examination however, can also be found in the presence of rather small volumes of pericardial effusion: if the heart is dilated for some reason, a small volume of pericardial fluid is already obstructive to inflow. Also, if elasticity of the pericardium is lost for some reason, a small volume of fluid is already obstructive. Consequently, the detection of inflow obstruction is more important than the estimation of the volume of pericardial effusion.

In most patients, the echo-free space is divided equally throughout the pericardial cavity. If not, fibrin layers between the epicardium and pericardium may be present, sometimes also resulting in pocket formation. This may be a problem in case of pericardiocenthesis.

Localized pericardial effusion can be found from the subcostal view in front of RA and RV. Sometimes, intracardiac malignancies may be the cause. Several patients with intracardiac malignancies have been sent for echocardiography only because of suspected pericardial effusion, without any suspicion of a malignancy. The echo gave the first clue to the presence of a malignancy.

Echocardiography is extremely helpful in directing pericardiocenthesis.

Indications for pericardiocenthesis are inflow obstruction to the heart, caused by effusion or the need for diagnostics.

To be investigated in pericardial effusion
echocardiography:
- number of millimeters of echo-free space, visualized and described from as many views as possible
- is the effusion equally divided?
- is fibrin present?
- if localized in front of the right atrium and the right ventricle (from the subcostal view): are there echo masses in the right atrium, possibly caused by malignant growth?
- diameters of the IVC during respiration (IVC view) (obstruction?)
- diameters of the LV during respiration (long axis view) (obstruction?)

Constrictive pericarditis

In constrictive pericarditis, distension of a usually thickened pericardium is impaired. The cause is pericarditis, complicated by adherence of the pericardium to the epicardium. It is possible that calcium deposits are found in the pericardium on the chest X-ray. A pericardial knock may be audible. As distension of the heart is impaired, the symptoms and clinical and echocardiographic findings are the same as for tamponade caused by pericardial effusion (Fig. 8-163).

With echocardiography, the epi-pericardial double layer is visible as one thickened layer. Dense echoes may be found from that area. However, compared to calcium deposits on the chest X-ray, the echocardiogram may be rather disappointing as dense echoes are not always found in this situation.

To be investigated in constrictive pericarditis
echocardiography:
- diameters of the IVC during respiration (IVC view) (obstruction?)
- diameters of the LV during respiration (long axis view) (obstruction?)

Pericardial cysts

Pericardial cysts are rather uncommon and typically located at the right side of the heart. They are filled with clear fluid and are not loculated. It is a congenital anomaly. Usually they do not give rise to symptoms; they are often discovered by an abnormality on the chest X-ray. Examples of a pericardial cyst are presented in Fig. 8-164 and 8-165.

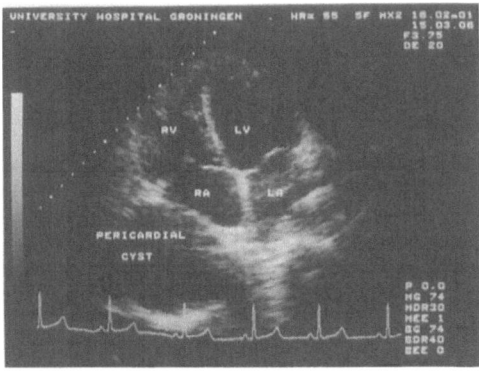

Fig. 8-164. Apical view of a pericardial cyst. A large echo-free space is found adjacent the RA.

CONGENITAL CARDIAC ABNORMALITIES IN THE ADULT

Many congenital cardiac abnormalities are known and can be diagnosed with echocardiography and Doppler. Only the abnormalities that are still commonly detected in the adult, are discussed in this Chapter. (Sub)valvular aortic stenosis is discussed in the section aortic valve, (sub)valvular pulmonic stenosis and double chambered RV are discussed in the section pulmonic valve.

Atrial septal defect and abnormal drainage of pulmonary veins

In atrial septal defect (ASD) a left-to-right shunt is usually found between the

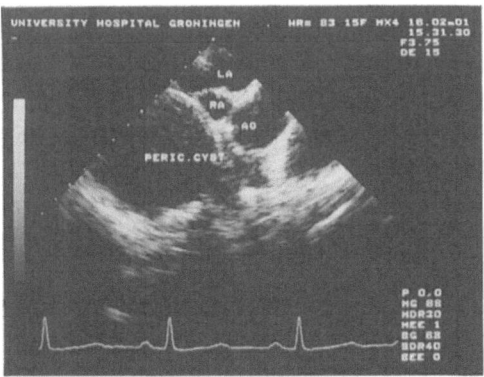

Fig. 8-165. TEE of the pericardial cyst (same patient as Fig. 8-164). In this section the RA is very small as it is displaced by the large cyst.

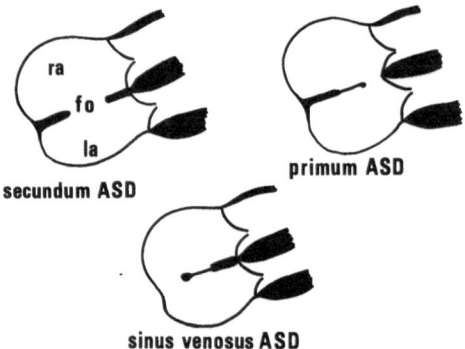

secundum ASD

primum ASD

sinus venosus ASD

Fig. 8-166. Types of ASD as can be visualized from the subcostal view. fo = fossa ovalis.

atria. However, in a small ASD also an isolated right-to-left shunt can be found.

There are three types of ASD: ASD type I (primum ASD), ASD type II (secundum ASD or fossa ovalis defect) and the sinus venosus type (Fig. 8-166).

All types have the same hemodynamic effects on the heart. These are also the same for abnormal drainage of pulmonary veins. In ASD type I or primum type ASD, the caudal part of the septum is absent. Usually, a cleft mitral valve is also found in combination with an ASD type I: minor or severe mitral insufficiency may be present. ASD type II is the most common type, being approximately 70% of all ASD's. In abnormal drainage, one or more pulmonary veins are connected to the RA instead of to the LA. There are a few more uncommon shunts at atrial level which are not further discussed here.

ASD results in a volume overload to the right heart. A fixed splitting of the second heart sound is typical, with a systolic pulmonic flow murmur, in larger shunts also with a diastolic tricuspid flow murmur. In abnormal venous drainage, the splitting of the second heart sound may be normal.

In larger shunts the ECG shows RV hypertrophy. The volume overload of the right heart may cause pulmonary hypertension. If RVEDP and RA pressure increase, the direction of the shunt may reverse. The patient then becomes cyanotic and dyspnoic.

Visualization of the defect

The normal inter-atrial septum is only partly visible from the apical view. The caudal and cranial parts can be identified but often the middle section is not seen. The direction of the ultrasound is parallel to this smooth structure (valvula fossa ovalis) and the ultrasound will not be reflected. The 'absence' of the middle part of the septum is almost always noticed from this view. How-

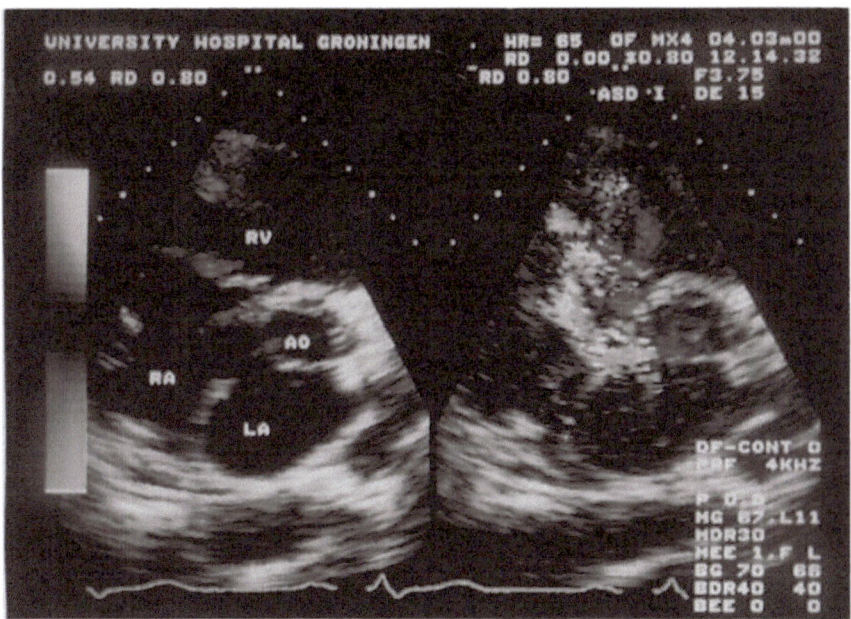

Fig. 8-167. ASD type I from the short axis aortic view. The ASD is diagnosed without color flow already (left). During atrial contraction a red color with aliasing enters the RA from the LA just below the aortic ring, proving an ASD type I. A very small shunt is also detected more apical in the RA as a very small area of red color that originates from the septum.

ever, occasionally, an ASD is suspected for the first time from the apical view: it may be present if a great change in diameter between apical and caudal parts of the inter-atrial septum is found during the cardiac cycle or an increased mobility of the septum. An enlarged RA then supports the diagnosis ASD.

In the short axis aortic view, the interpretation of an interruption of the septum is more reliable. The angle between ultrasound and septum is still small, but echoes are better as the septum is closer to the transducer. The position is also suitable for Doppler examinations (Fig. 8-167). The differentiation between the types of ASD is often possible from this view.

The angle between the ultrasound beams and the septum is about 70° from the subcostal view. This permits a reliable diagnosis of ASD. However, in many adults the quality of the subcostal recording is not good enough for evaluation. For visualization of the flow the subcostal view is less good than the short axis aortic view as the liver absorbs much of the color Doppler signals.

If Doppler is not available, contrast echocardiography may be helpful in the diagnosis (Chapter 4, 'contrast echocardiography').

Far the best view for the detection of an ASD is with TEE (Fig. 8-168). The inter-atrial septum is at a distance of about 3-4 cm from the transducer and is

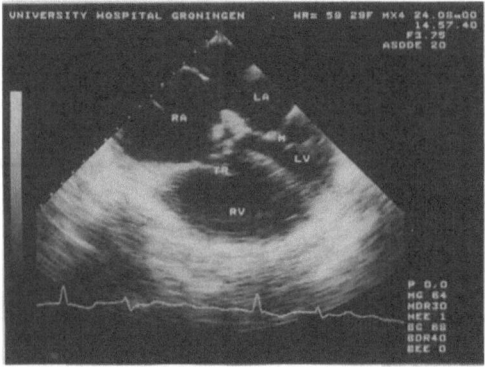

Fig. 8-168. TEE of an ASD type II. The inter-atrial septum is interrupted at the level of the fossa ovalis.

hit perpendicularly. The transducer position results in an excellent recording of the septum. It permits estimation of the size of the defect. In a small ASD with a left-to-right shunt the color flow is directed away from the transducer; if the shunt is from right to left it is towards the transducer (Fig.8-169, 8-170). The blue and turbulent colors from a left-to-right shunt should not be confused with the same colors from the flow, entering the RA via the SVC.

Effects on the heart

The volume overload, caused by shunting at atrial level, causes enlargement of the right heart. From the apical view, enlargement of the RA with respect with

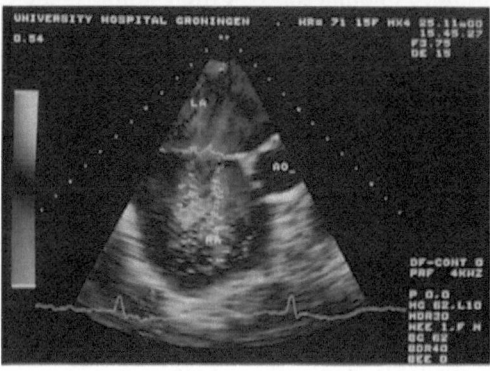

Fig. 8-169. TEE of an ASD type II. A blue color in the LA shows a direction of flow towards the inter-atrial septum. Aliasing is found at the level of the inter-atrial septum and below it. Turbulence is found deeper in the RA.

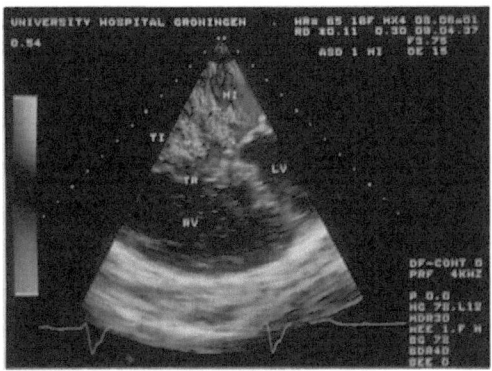

Fig. 8-170. TEE of an ASD type I. This systolic frame shows turbulent colors from tricuspid insufficiency (TI). The same is found from mitral insufficiency (MI) that originates from the AML from the area of the mitral ring. Both color areas mix at the level where the inter-atrial septum is absent. This proves an ASD type I with mitral insufficiency from a cleft mitral valve.

the LA is obvious. A second feature is the paradoxical septal motion pattern: the IVS moves towards the RV instead of towards the LV during systole. This is not specific to ASD and/or abnormal venous drainage. A paradoxical motion pattern can also be found in severe tricuspid regurgitation, severe pulmonic regurgitation and in pulmonary hypertension without RV volume overload.

In larger shunts trabecularization of the RV can be found, especially in the area of the apex. The RV wall may be thickened by hypertrophy.

Effects on the heart are further discussed in Chapter 8, 'Right ventricle'.

Contrast echocardiography

There is still a role for contrast echocardiography in the detection of an ASD. This is discussed in Chapter 4.

Doppler examinations

In most transducer positions, the flow through an ASD is perpendicular to the transducer. This results in good colors. The only proof using color for the presence of an ASD is when the color flow goes towards the inter-atrial septum, passes it and comes out of it. A false positive diagnosis is easily made if the flow only seems to originate from the inter-atrial septum. Especially with TEE, color flow analysis is ideal for the detection of multiple atrial septal defects. Pseudo pictures with color from ASD's are well known.

The flow velocity through the pulmonic valve is increased. Sometimes, the pulmonary-to-systemic flow ratio is calculated to estimate the severity of the shunt. Turbulent colors through the tricuspid valve can be found in moderate to severe shunting. Together with an enlarged RA this may be the only indication for the presence of a shunt at atrial level. Severe tricuspid insufficiency can mimic the situation, but this can easily be detected or excluded.

The pulmonary-to systemic flow ratio

The shunt severity can be established with the pulmonary-to-systemic flow ratio.

If outputs from RV and LV are determined with Doppler and also the cross sections of vessels, the pulmonary-to-systemic flow ratio can be determined. A ratio greater than 2.0 is considered significant. Good as well as poor correlations have been found with invasive methods. The principles of measurement of the cardiac output are described in Chapter 8, 'Left ventricle'.

To be investigated in ASD
echocardiography:
- great change in diameter of the inter-atrial septum? (apical view)
- paradoxical septal motion (long axis view)
- RA diameter (apical, subcostal view)
- RV size with respect to LV size (apical view)
- RV wall thickness (long axis view)
- visualization of the ASD? (subcostal view)
- localization of the ASD: which type?
- contrast-echocardiography: contrast in the LA after injection in a peripheral vein? (apical, subcostal view)
- cleft mitral valve in ASD I?
Doppler:
- (direction of) flow through the inter-atrial septum? (subcostal view)
- tricuspid insufficiency? (short axis aortic, apical, subcostal)
- mitral insufficiency in ASD I?
- severity of the shunt? (stroke volumes of RV and LV)
color Doppler:
- is the color going towards the atrial septum, does it pass it and does it come out of it?
- (direction of) flow through the atrial septum? (subcostal, apical view)
TEE:
- visualization of the defect
- visualization of the flow direction

To be excluded:
- severe tricuspid regurgitation (Doppler, liver pulse recording)
- severe pulmonic insufficiency (short axis aortic view, color Doppler)
- pulmonic stenosis (short axis aortic view with Doppler)
- pulmonary hypertension (short axis aortic, apical and/ subcostal view, CW Doppler and color Doppler)

Ventricular septal defect

The shunt through a small or moderate large VSD is usually from left to right. It is suspected by a loud systolic murmur in the parasternal region, often with a thrill. The patient usually has no complaints and a normal life expectancy. However, the defect has to be diagnosed, as there is a risk of endocarditis and the patient should be instructed concerning prophylaxis. In large VSD's, the patient may complain from dyspnea on exertion. If pulmonary hypertension develops the shunt can reverse and the patient becomes cyanotic and dyspnoic.

Most VSD's in the adult are located just below the aortic valve.

Echocardiography

A small VSD is usually not detected with echocardiography. Sometimes it can be seen from the parasternal view, which is also the best position for visualization of larger VSD's. The LA and LV may be enlarged in larger VSD's.

Doppler examinations

With Doppler, the severity of the shunt can be calculated theoretically. The principle of stroke volume measurement with Doppler and the diameters of the vessels is described in the section left ventricle. A special problem in this measurement is the turbulent flow through the VSD.

Color Doppler is an excellent tool for visualization of the flow and thus localization of the VSD and is ideal for the detection of multiple septal defects. From the parasternal views, a red color with aliasing and turbulence goes towards the IVS, passes it and enters the RV as a turbulant flow. The left-to-right shunt is present during systole but can also be present during diastole when the diastolic LV pressure is higher than the diastolic RV pressure (Fig. 8-171). A disturbed flow in the RV outflow tract can be found but this is not specific; it can also be caused by a double chambered RV and by infundibular pulmonic stenosis.

In a large VSD with pulmonary hypertension, a reversed flow may be found.

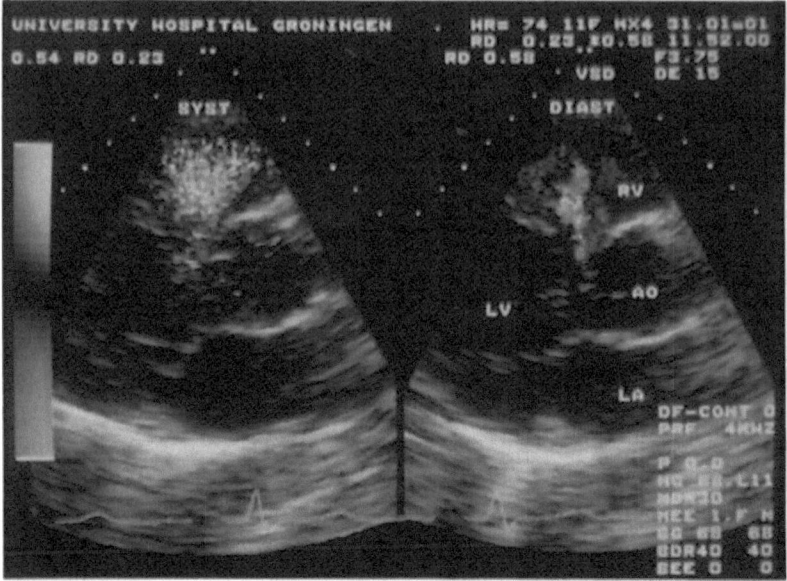

Fig. 8-171. Long axis view of a VSD. During systole a red color enters the IVS and passes it. The VSD causes turbulent colors in the RV. In this patient, the same flow -but without turbulence- is also seen during diastole, caused by an increased LV diastolic pressure.

Observation of the colors in the moving sector image may result in an incorrect diagnosis. The diastolic inflow into the RV mimics the systolic flow from a VSD. This is excluded easily by triggering the picture or by an M-mode recording.

Except for post-myocardial infarction VSD's, the apical transducer position is disappointing for visualization of the shunt with color: the flow is directed perpendicular to the transducer.

A small VSD is possibly a greater risk for endocarditis than a large VSD. Flow velocities through a small VSD are higher and damage of the endocardium is more likely then. In endocarditis, a ring of vegetations surrounds the VSD on the RV side. Satellite vegetations can be found on the opposite wall of the RV. The situation is often severe. Vegetations can be transported via the pulmonic valve to the lungs, causing severe pneumonia.

To be investigated in VSD
echocardiography:
– is interruption of the IVS visible? (parasternal long and short axis view)
– location(s) of the VSD?
Doppler:
– RV peak pressure (short axis aortic view)

– severity of the shunt? (stroke volumes from RV and LV)
color Doppler:
– is color flow going towards the IVS, does it pass the IVS and does it come out of it?
– direction(s) of shunting? (parasternal long and short axis view)

To be excluded (or also present)
– pulmonic stenosis
– sub-valvular pulmonic stenosis
– double chambered RV
– aortic insufficiency

Patent ductus arteriosus (Botalli)

In patent ductus arteriosus (PDA) a shunt is present from the aorta to the pulmonary artery. It is suspected or diagnosed by the presence of a continuous murmur at the first or second intercostal space at the left side of the sternum.

A PDA can be visualized from the short axis parasternal view and from the suprasternal view (Fig. 8-172). The flow can also be visualized with color Doppler from these positions.

Indirect evidence of the presence of a PDA is found from the continuous flow that can be detected in the pulmonary artery. The flow velocity through a ductus is maximal at end-systole.

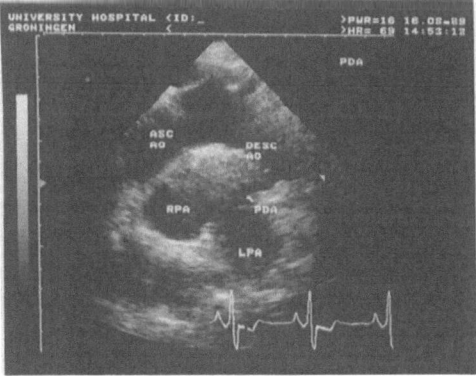

Fig. 8-172. Suprasternal view of a PDA. The ascending aorta (ASC AO), the aortic arch and the descending aorta (DESC AO) surround the right pulmonary artery (RPA). The PDA is visible as a connection between the pulmonary artery and the aorta. LPA = left pulmonary artery.

To be investigated in PDA
echocardiography:
– direct visualization (short axis parasternal and/or suprasternal view)
color:
– visualization of the flow (short axis parasternal and/or suprasternal view)

Ebstein's anomaly

Ebstein's anomaly is an abnormality of the tricuspid valve in which the septal leaflet inserts more apically along the IVS than normal. The anterior leaflet is elongated. The displacement of the septal leaflet results in 'atrialization' of part of the RV and a small functional RV. It is frequently associated with an ASD. Rhythm disturbances are common in these patients.

From the apical view the abnormal insertion can be detected easily. A displacement of more than 10 mm in the adult is indicative of Ebstein's anomaly (Fig. 8-173). A delay in tricuspid valve closure of 60-80 ms with respect to mitral valve closure can be detected with M-mode. This is not specific as it can also be found in RV volume overload.

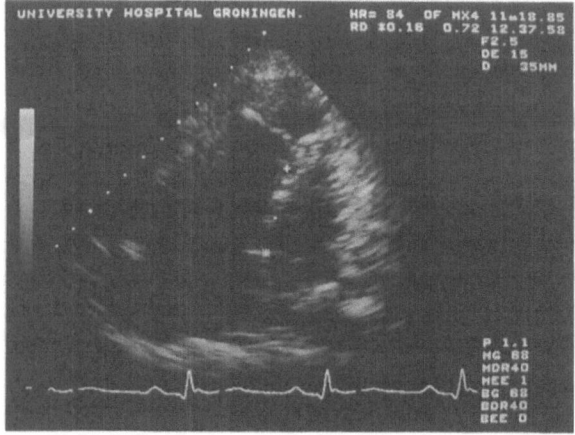

Fig. 8-173. Apical view of Ebstein's anomaly. The largest compartment is a combination of the RA and part of the RV (atrialized RV). The small RV is nearest to the transducer. The tricuspid valve is visible in the upper part of the image. The site of attachment to the IVS is indicated with +. The attachment of the mitral valve is indicated with *. The distance between both points is 35 mm which proves Ebstein's anomaly.

INTRACARDIAC MASSES

Echocardiography is the best technique for the detection of intracardiac and pericardial tumors. They are recorded as echo-masses of various echo-density and of various mobility.

As echocardiography fails to detect the microscopical nature of an echo-mass, only a probable diagnosis can be given. This is often possible with great reliability with help of other echocardiographic findings and with help of clinical and physical findings.

With the exclusion of vegetations, the differences between benign and malignant echo-masses are discussed in this Chapter.

Thrombi

Thrombi are usually not found in the normal heart. Low flow velocities in the heart as in dilated cardiomyopathy, favour thrombus formation. In enlarged atria, also in sinus rhythm, flow velocities are lower than normal and thrombus masses may be found there. In atrial fibrillation, when the atrial walls have little motion, thrombus masses are more likely to be present. This is especially so for the atrial appendages.

Thrombus masses are less often found in the ventricles. If located in the RV, they have to be differentiated from the moderator band. Emboli from peripheral veins can also be found in the RV as snake-like echo masses. Thrombus formation is more often found in the LV than in the RV: in myocardial infarction with lower flow velocities and akinetic parts of the LV wall, a thrombus can easily develop.

Thrombi often have the same echo-density as myocardium. Generally, thrombi in the atria are more or less oval in shape, with a smooth contour. They are broadly attached to the wall, often to the postero-lateral wall of the left atrium. Layered thrombi have also been found in the atria. Thrombi in the LV may have the same flattened appearances and are attached to an akinetic or hypokinetic part of the LV wall, usually in an enlarged LV with low flow velocities. Sometimes circular shaped, mobile thrombus masses are found in the LV (Fig. 8-174).

All possible echocardiographic views should be used to find or to exclude a thrombus. The best position for the detection of atrial thrombi is with TEE.

A patient with an intracardiac thrombus may have had symptoms of peripheral embolization. Also, many thrombi are found during echocardiographic examinations, performed for other reasons.

Most thrombi are immobile, but mobile thrombi have been described, especially from the right heart.

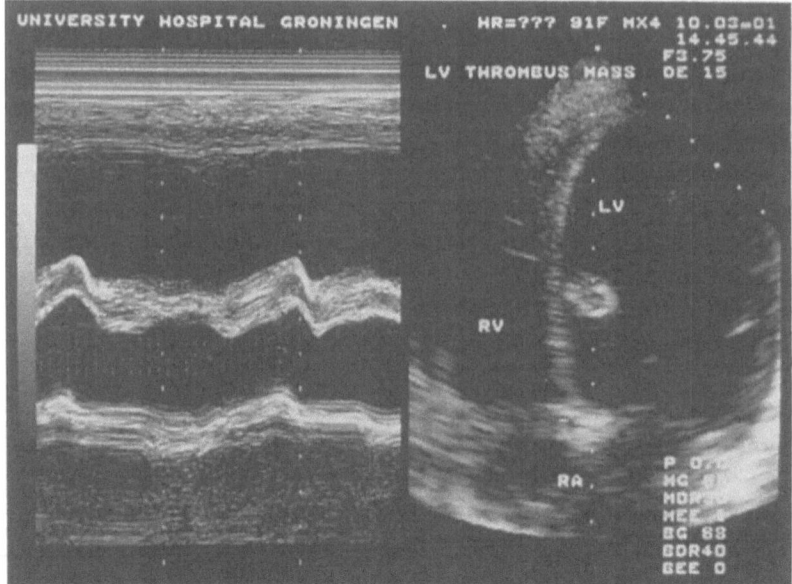

Fig. 8-174. Small thrombus at the mid-septal region of a poorly contracting dilated LV. The M-mode recording shows a rather good mobility of the thrombus.

Myxomas

The most common benign intracardiac tumor is a myxoma. About 75% of all myxomas is found in the LA, 25% in the RA. Occasionaly, a myxoma is found in the ventricles. As embolization often occurs, location of the myxoma in the LA is dangerous. Malignant degeneration has not been found until now.

The patient's complaints in myxoma may be caused by atrial rhythm disturbances, symptoms of mitral or tricuspid valve obstruction or results of embolization. Very often the temperature is subfebrile and the ESR moderately increased. Also, a patient may have no complaints from a myxoma, but has other complaints that were the reason for echocardiography. On physical examination the first heart sound is almost always very loud, irrespective of the consistency of the myxoma. Sometimes a tumor plop is heard, resembling a normal third heart sound. Depending on location and size, the same murmurs are audible as from mitral- or tricuspid stenosis. Also, mitral insufficiency murmurs are possible, caused only by the myxoma.

The typical appearance of a myxoma is a dense echo-mass of a loose consistency, attached to the inter-atrial septum and moving with the blood flow from LV to LA and backwards. A myxoma is usually attached with a small pedicle to the rim of the fossa ovalis (Fig. 8-175). The finding of a pedicle

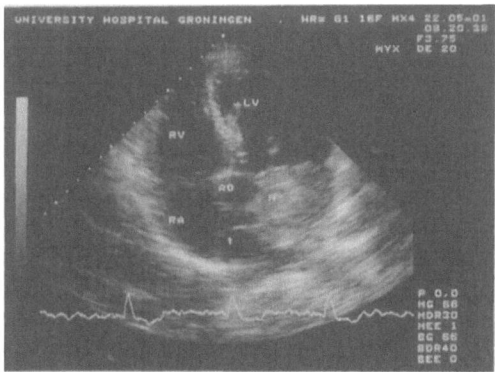

Fig. 8-175. Apical view of a LA myxoma (M). The attachment with a small pedicle (arrow) to the rim of the fossa ovalis almost proves a myxoma.

is almost a proof of a myxoma. As most myxomas are located in the LA, TEE is the superior technique for further evaluation (Fig. 8-176).

Exceptions to the high echo-density are known: sometimes the density is low and a myxoma can be missed with echocardiography when it is almost echo-translucent.

There are also exceptions to the site of attachment at the rim of the fossa ovalis. Myxomas can also be found attached more cranially at the inter-atrial septum and also at the roof of the LA. Occasionally, it is seen as an immobile, very echogenic mass attached to the inter-atrial septum, from which the attachment starts at the rim of the fossa ovalis and ends at the base of the anterior mitral leaflet: an attachment of $2^{1}/_{2}$ cm. Myxomas can also be attached

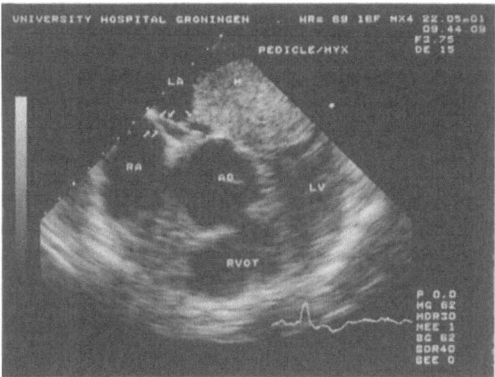

Fig. 8-176. TEE of a LA myxoma. The pedicle (single arrow) almost proves the nature of the echo mass.

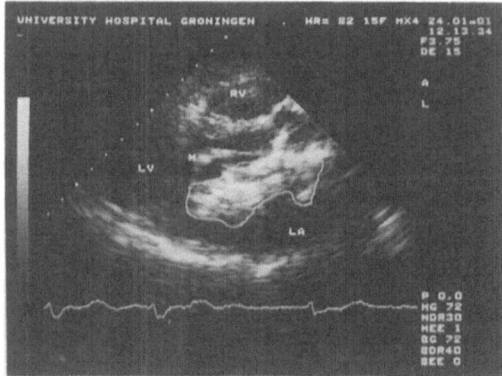

Fig. 8-177. Long axis view of an uncommon myxoma. The myxoma is stiff, immobile and extremely echogenic.

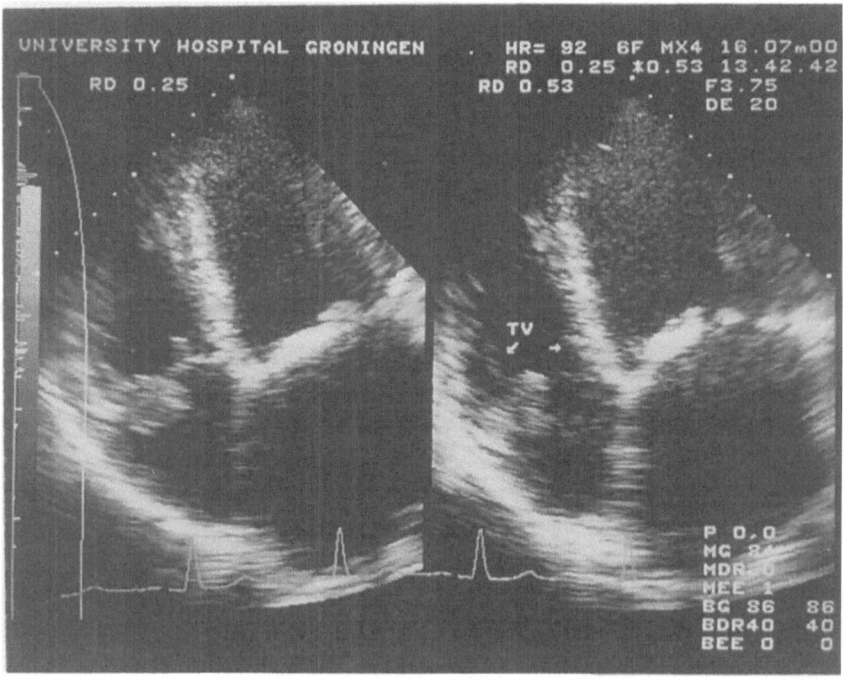

Fig. 8-178. Apical view of a myxoma, attached to the tricuspid leaflet. Two leaflets of the tricuspid valve (TV) are recorded during diastole (arrows). The difference in position of the echo mass proves attachment to the lateral tricuspid leaflet.

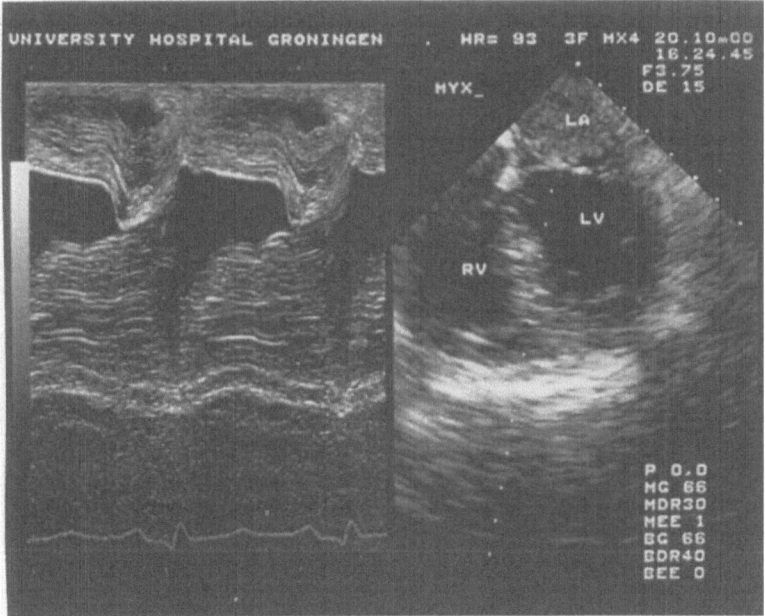

Fig. 8-179. TEE of a myxoma, attached to the AML.

to the tricuspid (Fig. 8-177, 8-178) and mitral valve (Fig. 8-179) without a pedicle. They should be differentiated from thrombi or vegetations: in fresh vegetations the patient has signs and symptoms of endocarditis; also, valve myxomas are usually not attached to the leading edges of the valve as is the case with vegetations. The valve myxomas are usually attached to the atrial side of the valves. If flow velocities are normal, it is unlikely that echo-masses attached to valves, are thrombi.

Exceptions to the loose consistency are also known: egg-shaped myxomas with a smooth surface have been found without a change in shape during the cardiac cycle.

Malignancies

Malignancies may involve the heart by direct extension of a pulmonic or mediastinal neoplasm. Occasionally, hematogenic metastases are found in the heart, for example from a malignant melanoma. More than one mass may be found then.

Direct invasion of the heart can be found into ventricular and atrial walls but is most often found in the RA and less often in the LA. The invaded myocardi-

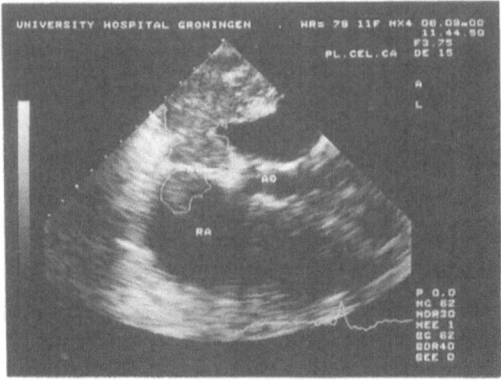

Fig. 8-180. TEE of a cardiac malignancy. The LA is almost filled up with an immobile echo mass that invades the inter-atrial septum (AS). The tracing of the mass shows extension into the RA. The mass is caused by a planocellular carcinoma of the lungs.

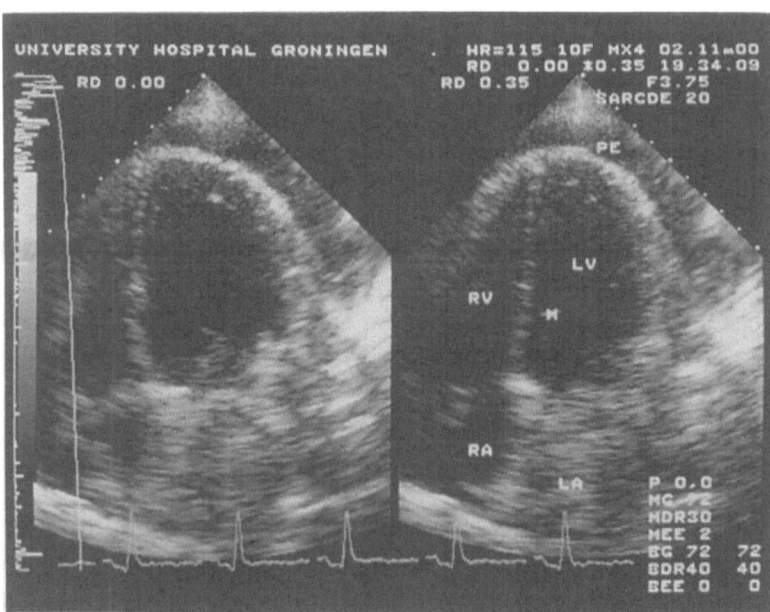

Fig. 8-181. Apical view of invasion of the LA and part of the LV by a solid, immobile mass with a broad attachment. The pericardial effusion (PE) supports the suspicion of a malignancy. The mass is caused by direct invasion of a bronchial carcinoma.

um is usually more echogenic than the surrounding normal myocardium. The motion from that particular part of the wall is impaired. Intra-cavitary echo masses can be found, attached to the lateral wall of the heart. Those masses are usually broadly attached, have a high echo-density and are immobile.

If an echo mass invades anatomic structures, it is highly suspicious for a malignancy (Fig. 8-180).

Pericardial effusion is often present in malignancies (Fig. 8-181); especially from the subcostal view several masses in combination with pericardial effusion can be detected which may be the first indication of a possible malignancy (Fig. 8-182). An echo-guided pericardiocenthesis should be performed to detect malignant cells.

Almost always, immobility and broad attachment favour a malignancy (Fig. 8-183).

Invasion of the heart via the IVC is also possible (Fig. 8-52) especially from a Grawitz tumor.

Questionable recordings

From the parasternal long axis view a high echo-density of the posterior part of the mitral ring may be confused with a thrombus or a malignancy. A malignancy is unlikely if a good shift between epi- and pericardium is recorded. This almost excludes direct growth into the heart. Also, from other transducer positions, including TEE, a mass can often be excluded. A comparable echo-

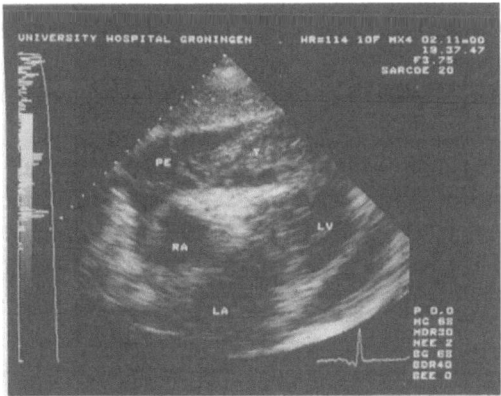

Fig. 8-182. Subcostal view of the same patient as Fig. 8-181. Much pericardial effusion (PE) is found in front of RA and RV, filled with structures (T) (tumor, fibrin?). An echogenic mass is found in the RA.

216

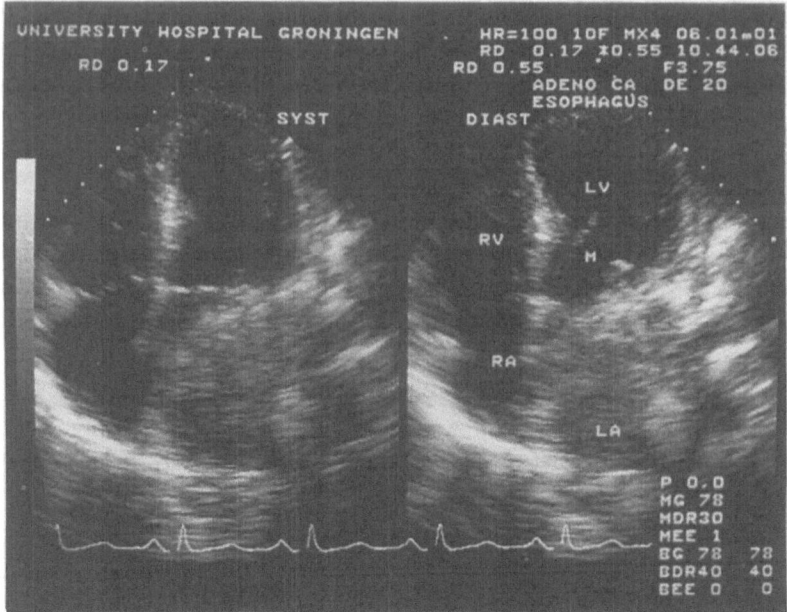

Fig. 8-183. Apical view of invasion of an adenocarcinoma of the esophagus in the LA. The mass is almost immobile and invades the LA wall.

genic mass is possible from the lateral part of the tricuspid ring (subcostal view, apical view). Also, if there is no pericardial effusion and if a good shift can be recorded between epi- and pericardium, a malignancy is not very likely to exist in that region.

From the subcostal transducer position, a partly thickened inter-atrial septum is not an uncommon finding. Usually only the caudal and less often the apical part is thickened and echogenic, caused by lipomatous infiltration. TEE is ideal for recording this.

With echocardiography, all transducer positions should be used before intracardiac masses are diagnosed or excluded; this includes the subcostal view. Especially for intra-atrial masses, TEE is almost indispensable: intra-atrial masses have frequently been detected with TEE, which were not found with TTE (Fig. 8-184, 8-185).

For the differentiation between benign and malignant echo masses
– LA location favours thrombus or myxoma
– RA location favours malignancy
– broad attachment favours malignancy, small attachment myxoma
– a pedicle to the rim of the fossa ovalis almost proves a myxoma

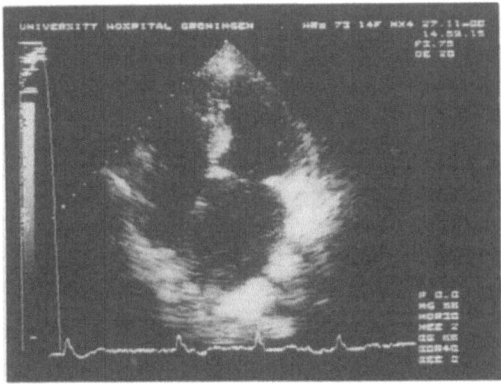

Fig. 8-184. Apical view of invasion of a non-Hodgkin lymphoma in RA and LA. Except for an enlarged LA, no obvious abnormalities are seen in this view.

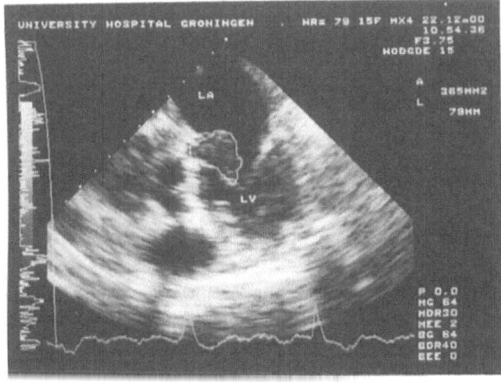

Fig. 8-185. TEE of the same patient as in Fig. 8-184. Besides the traced area at the AML, almost the whole RA is invaded with a mass that appeared to be a non Hodgkin lymphoma.

- invasement of natural structures almost proves a malignancy
- high mobility favours myxoma
- pericardial effusion favours malignancy
- a smooth surface favours thrombi
- local increased echo-density of a slightly thickened heart wall with impaired motion of the wall favours malignancy
- multiple echo-masses favour malignancies (hematogenic)
- high flow velocities do not favour thrombi

To be investigated in intracardiac masses
echocardiography:

- location in the heart
- multiple masses
- site of attachment
- broad or small attachment
- pedicle
- loose or solid consistency
- smooth or irregular surface
- mobility and change in shape during the cardiac cycle
- pericardial effusion
- at the site of attachment: is the echo-density of the myocardium stronger than normal?
- obstruction of the mass of a valve orifice
- size of the atria (rhythm)

Doppler:
- normal or low flow velocities

color Doppler:
- indirect evaluation of the size of the tumor, especially in echo-translucent tumors

TEE:
- same questions as above

References

Feigenbaum H: Echocardiography, 4th ed. Philadelphia, Lea & Febiger, 1986.

Hatle L, Angelson B: Doppler ultrasound in cardiology: physical principles and clinical applications, 2nd ed. Philadelphia, Lea & Febiger, 1984.

Chapman JV, Sgalambro A: Basic concepts in Doppler echocardiography. Dordrecht, Martinus Nijhoff Publishers, 1988.

Kisslo J, Adams DB, Belkin RN: Doppler color flow imaging. New York, Churchill Livingstone, 1988.

Nanda NC: Doppler echocardiography. New York Igaku-Shoin, 1985.

Popp RL, Fowles R, Coltart J, Martin RP: Cardiac anatomy viewed systematically with two-dimensional echocardiography. Chest 75:579, 1979.

Likoff M, Reichek N, St John Sutton M, Macoviak J, Harken A: Epicardial mapping of segmental myocardial function: an echocardiographic method applicable in man. Circulation 66:1050, 1982.

Ren JF et al: Effect of coronary bypass surgery and valve replacement of left ventricular function: assessment by intraoperative two-dimensional echocardiography. Am Heart J 109:281, 1985.

Popp RL, Filly K, Brown OR, Harrison DC: Effect of transducer placement and echocardiographic measurement of left ventricular dimensions. Am J Cardiol 35:537, 1975.

Fowles RE, Martin RP, Popp RL: Apparent asymmetric septal hypertrophy due to angled interventricular septum. Am J Cardiol 46:386, 1980.

Report of The American Society of Echocardiography Committee on Nomenclature and Standards: Identification of Myocardial Wall Segments, 1982.

Crawford MH, White DH, Amon KW: Echocardiographic evaluation of left ventricular size and performance during handgrip and supine and upright bycicle exercise. Circulation 59:1188, 1979.

Wann LS, Faris JV, Childress RH, Dillon JC, Weyman AE, Feigenbaum H: Exercise cross-sectional echocardiography in ischemic heart disease. Circulation 60:1300, 1979.

Visser CA, van der Wieken RL, Kan G, Lie KI, Busemann-Sokele, Meltzer RS, Durrer D: Comparison of two-dimensional echocardiography with radionuclide angiography during dynamic exercise for the detection of coronary artery disease. Am Heart J 106:528, 1983.

Pombo JF,Troy BL, Russell RO Jr: Left ventricular volumes and ejection fraction by echocardiography. Circulation 43:480, 1971.

Gibson DG: Measurement of left ventricular volumes in man by echocardiography-comparison with biplane angiographs. Br Heart J 33:614, 1971.

Teichholz LE, Kreulen T, Herman MV, Gorlin R: Problems in echocardiographic volume determinations: Echocardiographic-angiographic correlations in the presence or absence of asynergy. Am J Cardiol 37:7, 1976.

Upton MT, Gibson DG, Brown DJ: Echocardiographic assessment of abnormal left ventricular relaxation in man. Br Heart J 38:1001, 1976.

Stamm RB, Carabello BA, Mayers DL, Martin RP: Two-dimensional echocardiographic measurement of left ventricular ejection fraction: Prospective analysis of what constitutes an adequate determination. Am Heart J 104:136, 1982.

Gardin JM, Iseri LT, Elkayam U, Tobis J, Childs W, Burn CS, Henry WL: Evaluation of dilated cardiomyopathy by pulsed Doppler echocardiography. Am Heart J 106:1057, 1983.

Maron BJ, Spirito P, Green KJ, Wesley YE, Bonow RO, Arce J: Noninvasive assessment of left ventricular diastolic function by pulsed Doppler echocardiography in patients with hypertrophic cardiomyopathy. JACC 10-4:733, 1987.

Bryg RJ, Pearson AC, Williams GA, Labovitz AJ: Left ventricular systolic and diastolic flow abnormalities determined by Doppler echocardiography in obstructive hypertrophic cardiomyopathy. AJC 59:925, 1987.

Oda H: Left ventricular responses to dopamine in dilated cardiomyopathy as assessed by two-dimensional echocardiography and compared with findings of thallium-201 scintigraphy. Tohoku J exp Med, 153 (3):217, 1987.

Dragalescu SI, Streian C, Cristodorescu R, Stoichescu L: Echocardiographic approach to the early diagnosis of congestive cardiomyopathies. Med Interne 22 (3):179 1984,

Staiger J, Simon G, Pauer A, Keul J: Echokardiographische Kontraktilitätsreserve unter körperlicher Belastung bei Herzgesunden und Patienten mit dilatativer Kardiomyopathie. Ztschr für Kardiologie 76(10):635, 1987.

Borow KM, Lang RM, Neumann A, Caroll JD, Rajfer SI: Physiologic mechanisms governing hemodynamic responses to positive inotropic therapy in patients with dilated cardiomyopathy. Circulation 77 (3):625, 1988.

Gaasch WH: Left ventricular radius to wall thickness ratio. Am J Cardiol 43:1189, 1979.

Dittman H, Voelker W, Karsch KR, Seipel L: Vergleich Doppler-echokardiographischer Methoden zur Herzminutenvolumenbestimmung. Ztschr fur Kardiologie 76,7:433, 1987.

Takenaka K, Dabestani A, Gardin JM, Russell D, Clark S, Henry WL: Pulsed Doppler Echocardiographic study of left ventricular filling in dilated cardiomyopathy. Am J Cardiol 58:143, 1986.

Kronik G, Slany J, Mösslacher H: Comparitive value of eight M-mode echocardiographic formulas for determining left ventricular stroke volume. Circulation 60,6:1308, 1979.

Gardin JM, Iseri LT, Elkayam U, Tobis J, Childs W, Burn CS, Henry WL: Evaluation of dilated cardiomyopathy by pulsed Doppler echocardiography. Am Heart J 106,5,1:1057, 1983.

Nishimura RA, Callahan MJ, Schaff HV, Ilstrup DM, Miller FA, Tajik AJ: Non-invasive measurement of cardiac output by continuous wave Doppler echocardiography: Initial experience and review of the literature. Mayo Clin Proc 59:484, 1984.

Pratt RC, Parisi AF, Harrington JJ, Sasahara AA: The influence of left ventricular stroke volume on aortic root motion: An echocardiographic study. Circulation 53:947, 1976.

Ambrose J, Martinez E, Teichholz L, Meller J, Pichard A, Herman M: The slope of the posterior aortic root during atrial systole-an index of left ventricular chamber stiffness. Curculation (Suppl II) 60:121, 1979 (Abstract).

Hamer JPM: Problems and pitfalls in the diagnosis of hypertrophic cardiomyopathy. In: Recent views on hypertrophic cardiomyopathy. Dordrecht, Martinus Nijhoff, 1985.

Visser CA: Two-dimensional echocardiography in acute and chronic myocardial infarction. Amsterdam, 1982.

Delemarre BJM: Doppler echocardiography in coronary artery disease. Amsterdam, Weka, 1987.

Koolen JJ: Left ventricular monitoring by transesophageal echocardiography. Amsterdam, 1987.

Hanrath P, Bleifeld W, Souquet J: Cardiovascular diagnosis by ultrasound. Transesophageal, computerized, contrast, Doppler echocardiography. The Hague, Martinus Nijhoff Publishers, 1982.

Visser CA, Kan G, Becker AE, Durrer D: Apex two dimensional echocardiography. Alternative approach to quantification of acute myocardial infarction. Br Heart J 47:461, 1982.

Visser CA, Durrer D: Echocardiographic determination of infarct size in acute myocardial infarction. Pract Cardiol 9:225, 1983.

Reeder GS, Seward JB, Tajik AJ: The role of two dimensional echocardiography in coronary artery disease. Mayo Clin Proc 57:247, 1982.

Bommer W, Weinert L, Nemann A, Neef j, Mason DT, DeMaria A: Determination of right atrial and right ventricular size by two-dimensional echocardiography. Circulation 60:91, 1979.

Nanda NC, Gramiak R, Robinson TI, Shah PH: Echocardiographic evaluation of pulmonary hypertension. Circulation 50:575, 1974.

Skjaerpe T, Hatle L: Noninvasive estimation of systolic pressure in the right ventricle in patients with tricuspid regurgitation. Eur Heart J 7:704, 1986.

Martin-Duran R, Larman M, Trugeda A, Vazquez de Prada JA, Ruano J, Torres A, Figueroa A, Pajaron A, Nistal F: Comparison of Doppler-determined increased pulmonary arterial pressure measured at cardiac catheterization. Am J Cardiol 57:859, 1986.

Dabestani A, Mahan G, Gardin JM, Takenaka K, Burn C, Allfie A, Henry WL: Evaluation of pulmonary artery pressure and resistance by pulsed Doppler echocardiography. Am J Cardiol 59:662, 1987.

Hamer JPM, Takens BL, Posma JL, Lie KI: Noninvasive measurement of right ventricular systolic pressure by combined color-coded and continuous-wave Doppler ultrasound. Am J Cardiol 61:668, 1988.

Strunk BL, Fitzgerald JW, Lipton M, Popp RL, Barry WH: The posterior aortic wall echocardiogram: Its relationship to left atrial volume change. Circulation 54:744, 1976.

Cloez JL, Neimann JL, Chivoret G, Danchin N, Bruntz JF, Godenir JP, Faivre G: Echocardiographic rediscovery of an anatomical structure: The Chiari network. Apropos of 16 cases. Arch Mal Coeur 76:1284, 1983.

Bommer W, Weinert L, Neumann A, Neef J, Mason DT, deMaria A: Determination of right atrial and right ventricular size by two-dimensional echocardiography. Circulation 60:91, 1979.

O'Rourke RA: Value of Doppler echocardiography for quantifying valvular stenosis or regurgitation. Circulation 78 (2):483, 1988.

Hatle L, Angelson B, Tromsdal A: Noninvasive assessment of aortic stenosis by Doppler ultrasound. Br Heart J 43:284, 1979.

Berger M, Berdoff RL, Gallerstein PE, Goldberg E: Evaluation of aortic stenosis by continuous wave Doppler ultrasound. J Am Coll Cardiol 3:150, 1984.

Moene RJ: Systolic time intervals in congenital aortic stenosis. Amsterdam, Mondeel, 1974.

Cromme-Dijkhuis AH: Echocardiographic evaluation of congenital aortic stenosis in children and adolescents. Groningen, Universiteitsdrukkerij, 1987.

Labovitz AJ, Ferrara RP, Kern MJ, Bryg RJ, Mrosek DG, Williams GA: Quantitative evaluation of aortic insufficiency by continuous wave Doppler echocardiography. JACC 8 (6):1341, 1986.

Oh JK, Taliercio CP, Holmes DR, Reeder GS, Bailey KR, Seward JB, Tajik AJ: Prediction of the severity of aortic stenosis by Doppler aortic valve area determination: prospective Doppler-catheterization correlation in 100 patients. JACC 11:1227, 1988.

Fan PH, Kapur KK, Nanda NC: Color-guided Doppler echocardiographic assessment of aortic valve stenosis. JACC 12:441, 1988.

Ren JF, Kotler MN, DePace NL, Mintz GS, Kimbiris D, Kalman P, Ross J: Two-dimensional echocardiographic determination of left atrial emptying volume: A non-invasive index in quantifying the degree of nonrheumatic mitral regurgitation. J Am Coll Cardiol 2:729, 1983.

Douglas PS, Berko BA, Ioli A, Reichek N: Variable responses of mitral valve motion and flow in systemic hypertension and idiopathic dilated cardiomyopathy. Am J Cardiol 60:363, 1987.

Hamer JPM: Chordal rupture of the mitral valve: reappraisal of the diagnosis and treatment. Van Denderen, Groningen, 1984.

Jeresaty RM: Mitral valve prolapse. New York, Raven Press, 1979.

Hatle L, Brubakk A, Tromsdal A, Angelson B: Noninvasive assessment of pressure drop in mitral stenosis by Doppler ultrasound. Br Heart J 40:131, 1978.

Teichholz L, Caputo G, Ambrose J, Knopsler B, Martinez E, Herman M: First derivative of diastolic aortic root motion as a measure of transmitral flow. Am J Cardiol 45:436, 1980 (Abstract).

Wranne B, Ask P, Loyd D: Assessment of severity of mitral stenosis: a theoretical and experimental study with emphasis on the validity of the gradient half time (abstr). Proceedings of the Second International Congress on Cardiac Doppler. Kyoto, 85, 1986.

Karp K, Teien D, Bjerle P, Eriksson P: Reassessment of valve area determinations in mitral stenosis by the pressure half-time method: impact of left ventricular stiffness and peak diastolic pressure difference. J Am Coll Cardiol 13::594, 1989.

Wilkins GT, Weyman AE, Abascal VM, Block PC, Palacios IF: Percutaneous balloon dilatation of the mitral valve: an analysis of echocardiographic variables related to outcome and the mechanism of dilatation. Br Heart J 60:299, 1988.

Krivokapich J, Child JS, Dadourian BJ, Perlott JK: Reassessment of echocardiographic criteria for diagnosis of mitral valve prolapse. AJC 61:131, 1988.

Marino P, Zanolla L, Nidasio GP, Nicolosi GL, Fabbri A: Interpretative reproducibility of two-dimensional echocardiographic images. Analysis of intraobserver, interobserver and beat-to-beat reproducibility of the mitral orifice. Eur Heart J 4:733, 1983.

Glover MU, Warren SE, Vieweg WVR, Ceretto WJ, Samtoy LM, Hagan AD: M-mode and two-dimensional echocardiographic correlation with findings at catheterization and surgery in patients with mitral stenosis. Am Heart J 105:98, 1983.

Veyrat C, Ameur A, Bas S, Lessana A, Abitbol C, Kalmanson D: Pulsed Doppler echocardiographic indices for assessing mitral regurgitation. Br Heart J 51:130, 1984.

Barron JT, Manrose DL, Liebson PR: Comparison of auscultation with two-dimensional and Doppler echocardiography in patients with suspected mitral valve prolapse. Clin Cardiol 11:401, 1988.

Keren G, Katz S, Strom J, Sonnenblick EH, LeJemtel TH: Noninvasive quantification of mitral regurgitation in dilated cardiomyopathy: correlation of two Doppler echocardiographic methods. Am Heart J 116:758, 1988.

Weyman AE, Dillon JC, Feigenbaum H, Chang S: Echocardiographic patterns of pulmonic valve motion in pulmonic stenosis. Am J Cardiol 34:644, 1974.

222

Hoorntje JCA: Valvular pulmonic stenosis. Van Denderen, Groningen, 1987.

Ferrans VJ, Roberts WC: The carcinoid endocardial plaque. An ultrastructural study. Hum Pathol 7:387, 1976.

Lundin L, Norheim I, Landelius J, Oberg K, Theodorsson-Norheim E: Carcinoid heart disease: relationship of circulating vasoactive substances to ultrasound detectable cardiac abnormalities. Circulation 77:264, 1988.

Ferrans VJ, Roberts WC: The carcinoid endocardial plaque. An ultrastructural study. Hum Pathol 7:387, 1976.

Ramirez ML, Wong M, Sadler N, Shah PM: Doppler evaluation of bioprosthetic and mechanical aortic valves: data from four models in 107 stable, ambulatory patients. AHJ 115:418, 1988.

Rothbart RM, Smucker ML, Gibson RS: Overestimation by Doppler echocardiography of pressure gradients across Starr-Edwards prosthetic valves in the aortic position. AJC 61:475, 1988.

Dittrich H, Nicod P, Hoit B, Dalton N, Sahn D: Evaluation of Björk-Shiley prosthetic valves by real-time two-dimensional echocardiographic flow mapping. Am Heart J 115:133, 1988.

Nellessen U, Schnittger I, Appleton CP, Masuyama T, Bolger A, Fischell TA, Tye T, Popp RL: Transesophageal two-dimensional echocardiography and color Doppler flow velocity mapping in the evaluation of cardiac valve prostheses. Circulation 78:848, 1988.

Erbel R, Börner N, Steller D, Brunier J, Thelen M, Pfeiffer C, Mohr-Kahaly S, Iversen S, Oelert H, Meyer J: Detection of aortic dissection by transesophageal echocardiography. Br Heart J 58:45, 1987.

Cooke JP, Safford RE: Progress in the diagnosis and management of aortic dissection. Mayo Clin Proc 61:147, 1986.

Erbel R, Rohmann S, Drexler M, Mohr-Kahaly S, Gerharz CD, Iversen S, Oelert H, Meyer J: Improved diagnostic value of echocardiography in patients with infective endocarditis by transesophageal approach. A prospective study. Eur Heart J 9:43, 1988.

Wann LS, Dillon JC, Weyman AE, Feigenbaum H: Echocardiography in bacterial endocarditis. N Engl J Med 295:135, 1976.

Pandian NG, Brockway B, Simonetti J, Rosenfield K, Bojar RM, Cleveland RJ: Pericardiocentesis under two-dimensional echocardiographic guidance in located pericardial effusion. Ann Thorac Surg 45:99, 1988.

Tei C, Tanaka T, Nakao S, Tahara M, Kanehisa T: Echocardiographic analysis of interatrial septal motion. Am J Cardiol 44:472, 1979.

Hanrath P, Schluter M, Langenstein BA, Polster J, Engel S, Kremer P, Krebber HJ: Detection of ostium secundum atrial septal defects by transesophageal cross-sectional echocardiography. Br Heart J 49:350, 1983.

van Mill GJ, Moulaert AJ, Harinck E: Atlas of two-dimensional echocardiography in congential cardiac defects. The Hague, Martinus Nijhoff Publishers, 1983.

Oostman-Smith I, Silverman NH, Oldershow P, Lincoln C, Shinebourne EA: Cor triatriatum sinistrum. Diagnostic features on cross sectional echocardiography. Br Heart J 51:211, 1984.

Gussenhoven WJ, Jansen JRC, Bom N, Ligtvoet CM: Variability in the time interval between tricuspid and mitral valve closure in Ebstein's anomaly. J Clin Ultrasound 12:267, 1984.

Shiina A, Seward JB, Edwards WD, Hagler DJ, Tajik AJ: Two-dimensional echocardiographic spectrum of Ebstein's anomaly: detailed anatomic assessment. J Am Coll Cardiol 3:356, 1984.

Radford DJ, Graff RF, Neilson GH: Diagnosis and natural history of Ebstein's anomaly. Br Heart J 54:517, 1985.

Pollick C, Sullivan H, Cujec B, Wilansky S: Doppler color-flow imaging assessment of shunt size in atrial septal defect. Circulation 78 (3):522, 1988.

Werner JA, Cheitlin MD, Gross BW, Speck SM, Ivey TD: Echocardiographic appearance of the Chiari network: differentiation from right-heart pathology. Circulation 63:1104, 1981.

McAllister HA, Fenoglio JJ: Tumors of the cardiovascular system. Washington, Armed Forces Insitute of Pathology, 1978.

Chapter 9. The echocardiographic report

An echocardiographic report should be useful and reliable in clinical decision making. It is reliable if measurements were made carefully with a description of the quality of the recordings and, as far as possible, an echocardiographic differential diagnosis.

A question is formulated before echocardiography is performed and an answer to that question should be given. However, the question itself may be poor. For example, the question 'Is endocarditis present?': vegetation-like structures may be found, but if they are not detected, endocarditis still may be present. Such remarks should be mentioned in the report.

The quality and reliability of signals must be reported. This may not only be vital to the patient but also to the echocardiographer. For example, the CW Doppler signals from aortic stenosis may be clear or they may be difficult to record and measure and thus less reliable. In the authors institute the value of such comments were checked over a two year period. The measurements reported as 'clear and reliable signals' had excellent correlations with the findings at cardiac catheterization, whereas comments such as 'difficult to measure', or 'poor quality recording' had a less good correlation. Such comments are not only useful for decision making, but also may save the credibility of the echocardiographer.

It should always be remembered that an echocardiograph is not a microscope. Consequently, a comment like 'thrombus mass in the LA' cannot be made since the examiner cannot be sure about the origin of the mass of echoes. The echo mass may have been caused by other abnormalities. In such cases a differential diagnosis should be given with a description of the recordings from which the most likely diagnosis can be concluded. For example, a better comment would be 'mass of echoes in the LA, most likely a thrombus'.

Another example of an incorrect conclusion is 'aortic stenosis' if only made from an obviously calcified aortic valve with a poor motion pattern and a poor leaflet separation. Such a conclusion should not be made. Indirect features of aortic stenosis may be present from e.g. the LV wall thickness, but the diagnosis and the severity can only be verified from a good quality Doppler recording.

Values of pressure differences depend on many factors, of which the heart rate is very important. All pressure differences are zero if the heart rate is zero! Consequently, for each measurement of a pressure difference, the heart rate at the moment of measurement should be reported.

Every institution uses its own type of report and the layout of a report depends on the demands and interests of that specific institution. In many cases the report is stored in a computer. Almost all items of the report can be coded, but a conclusive description should always be made and is not codeble.

Example of an echocardiographic report.
   patients ID:

   date:

   name of examiner:

   quality of the recordings: good/rather good/poor

   Measurements:
- septal thickness
   excursion (long axis view)
- LVPW thickness
   excursion (long axis view)
- LV systolic/diastolic (long axis)
- LA diameters (long axis/apical)
- RA diameter (apical)
- IVC diameters inspiration/expiration
Measurements, important for the specific abnormality
for example:
in aortic insufficiency
- diameter of the aortic root
- a/H ratio from the apexcardiogram
in aortic stenosis
- CW Doppler measurement
Descriptive report:
- IVS and LVPW thickening during systole
- motion pattern of the LV local/diffuse hyper-/hypo-/akinesis
- RV size with respect to LV size (apical view)
- have measurements of pressure differences been made with or without
   correction for the angle?

- a (differential) diagnosis
- the severity of the abnormality
- other abnormalities that are excluded

Tracings of LV 'volumes' can also be computerized as are many other echocardiographic and Doppler measurements.

Documentation

Recordings from which measurements are made should be filed. It allows interpretation of measurements, made at follow-up examinations. These may be M-mode recordings or frozen pictures from sector images or computerized tracings.

The best method for recording the examination is on video. However, this requires many tapes and the space required is not always available. The choice made will vary between institutions.

Chapter 10. Anatomy, nomenclature and function of the normal heart

Anatomy and nomenclature of the normal heart

The heart consists of four cavities, separated from each other by walls and valves. The blood enters the heart in the right atrium via the superior vena cava (upper part of the body) and the inferior vena cava (lower part of the body). Both vessels have no valves. The wall of the right atrium is only a few millimeters thick. The right atrium is separated from the right ventricle by the tricuspid ring (annulus) and -valve. The ring consists of fibrous tissue. The tricuspid valve has three leaflets, the anterior, the posterior and the medial (or septal) leaflet which are connected to the papillary muscles with a number of chordae tendinae. The papillary muscles are part of the right ventricular wall. The right ventricle partly surrounds the left ventricle and ends in the right ventricular outflow tract at the pulmonic valve. The pulmonic valve consists of three cusps, the anterior, the right and the left cusp. The blood then passes through the pulmonary artery via the main branches, the right and left pulmonary artery.

After leaving the lungs, the blood enters the left atrium via the pulmonary veins. The left atrium is separated from the right atrium by the inter-atrial septum from which before birth, the fossa ovalis permitted the blood to go from the right atrium to the left atrium. This ostium is closed after birth by the valvula fossa ovalis.

The shape and anatomy of the left atrium is similar to the right atrium. The mitral valve is found between left atrium and left ventricle. The valve is one of the six components of the mitral apparatus. This consists of the left atrium, the mitral ring, the mitral valve, the chordae, the papillary muscles and the left ventricular wall. The function of the mitral apparatus depends on the integrity of these components. The valve is the only cardiac valve with two leaflets. The anterior leaflet is the largest one (longer), but occupies the smallest part of the mitral ring. The posterior leaflet is the smaller one (shorter), but occupies the major part of the mitral ring. The posterior leaflet usually consists of three functional entities. The chordae are attached to the leading edges of the leaflets and on the leaflets, a few milimeters from the edges. They end in two groups of papillary muscles, the anteromedial and the posterolateral papillary muscles.

The left ventricle is ovally shaped and has the thickest wall of all heart cavities. It ends in the left ventricular outflow tract with the aortic valve. Like the pulmonic valve, the aortic valve consists of three cusps, the right-, left- and non-coronary cusp. Each cusp creates a sinus of Valsalva. From the antero-posterior view, the aortic valve is located behind the pulmonic valve. The ascending aorta is in front of the pulmonic artery and is followed by the aortic arch and the descending thoracic aorta. The aortic arch 'hangs' over the right pulmonary artery with both vessels perpendicular to each other.

Function of the normal heart

Function of the right atrium

The function of the right atrium is to collect venous blood from the superior vena cava and inferior vena cava for transportation towards the right ventricle. The blood enters the right atrium by several factors from which inspiration and the downward motion of the tricuspid valve ring during ventricular systole should be mentioned.

During inspiration the intrathoracic pressure decreases which causes blood to enter the chest via the SVC and IVC. This is visible from the neck veins as well as from the collapse of the IVC with echocardiography. The blood gathers in the right atrium. Most of the blood enters the right ventricle by its relaxation, only a small part of it is transported actively by atrial contraction.

The contraction of the right ventricle causes opening of the pulmonic valve and transportation of the blood towards the lungs where it is oxygenated. As the lungs have less resistance to the heart than to the whole body, the right ventricle has less work to do than the left ventricle. Consequently, its wall is much thinner. After leaving the lungs, the blood enters the left atrium.

The left atrium collects blood from the lungs for transportation to the left ventricle. As functions of both atria are rather passive and they are both separated from the ventricles during systole, pressures in left and right atrium are low and almost the same.

Most of the blood from the pulmonary veins enters the left atrium during ventricular contraction by downward motion of the mitral ring. The blood is collected in the left atrium and kept ready for further transportation to the left ventricle. From the total left atrial volume only a part is ejected into the left ventricle. The left atrial volume decreases largely due to passive filling of the left ventricle. Almost 75% of the end-diastolic volume of the left ventricle is obtained by passive filling, 25% by active transportation by atrial contraction.

The left ventricle pumps the blood all through the body except for the lungs. Consequently, the pressure in the left ventricle is higher than in the right ventricle and its wall is thicker. Its contraction causes closure of the mitral valve and a short time later opening of the aortic valve.

The stroke volume is the volume of blood ejected during one ventricular contraction.

Cardiac output is the volume of blood ejected in one minute, i.e. stroke volume x heart rate.

The ejection fraction is that part of the end-diastolic volume that is ejected during ventricular systole.

Abbreviations

ACG	apexcardiogram
AML	anterior mitral leaflet
ASD	atrial septal defect
CW	continuous wave Doppler
DCM	dilating cardiomyopathy
ECG	electrocardiogram
ETI	ejection time index
HCM	hypertrophic cardiomyopathy
HOCM	hypertrophic obstructive cardiomyopathy
IVC	inferior vena cava
IVCT	isovolumic contraction time
IVRT	isovolumic relaxation time
IVS	interventricular septum
LA	left atrium
LV	left ventricle
LVEDP	left ventricular end-diastolic pressure
LVET	left ventricular ejection time
LVPW	left ventricular posterior wall
PEP	pre-ejection period
PD	pulsed Doppler
PDA	persistant ductus arteriosus (Botalli)
PML	posterior mitral leaflet
PRF	pulse repetetion frequency
Q-IIA	electromechanical interval
RA	right atrium
RV	right ventricle
RVEDP	right ventricular end-diastolic pressure
SVC	superior vena cava
TEE	trans-esophageal echocardiography
TI	tricuspid insufficiency
TTE	trans-thoracic echocardiography
VSD	ventricular septal defect

Index

Developments in Cardiovascular Medicine

Developments in Cardiovascular Medicine